FOOD VALUES
Fiber

OTHER BOOKS IN THE FOOD VALUES SERIES

Food Values: Calcium
Food Values: Calories
Food Values: Carbohydrates
Food Values: Cholesterol and Fats
Food Values: Sodium

FOOD VALUES

Fiber

Patty Bryan

PERENNIAL LIBRARY

Harper & Row, Publishers, New York

Grand Rapids, Philadelphia, St. Louis, San Francisco
London, Singapore, Sydney, Tokyo, Toronto

FIRST EDITION

Designed by Alma Orenstein

Library of Congress Cataloging-in-Publication Data

Bryan, Patty.
    Food values : fiber / Patty Bryan. — 1st ed.
        p.   cm.
    ISBN 0-06-096445-6
    1. Food—Fiber content—Tables. 2. Fiber in human nutrition. I. Title.
TX553.F53B79   1990
641.1—dc20   89-45633

90 91 92 93 94 AG/BC 10 9 8 7 6 5 4 3 2 1

Contents

Acknowledgments   vii

Introduction   ix

How to Use This Book   xv

Sources   xix

Abbreviations   xx

Baking Ingredients   1

Baking Mixes   1

Beef, Fresh & Cured   2

Beverages   2

Breadcrumbs, Croutons, Stuffings, & Seasoned
    Coatings   6

Breads, Rolls, Biscuits, & Muffins   6

Breakfast Cereals, Cold & Hot   8

Breakfast Foods, Prepared   19

Butter   20

Candy   20

Cheese & Cheese Foods   22

Cookies, Bars, & Brownies   22

Crackers   24

Desserts: Cakes, Pastries, & Pies   25

Desserts: Custards, Gelatins, & Puddings   26

Desserts, Frozen   27

Eggs & Egg Substitutes   27

Entrees & Main Courses, Canned   28

Fast Foods   28

Fats, Oils, & Shortenings   29

Flours & Cornmeal   29

Fruit, Fresh & Processed   31

Fruit Spreads   41

Infant & Toddler Foods   43

Lamb, Veal, & Miscellaneous Meats   56

Legumes & Legume Products   57

Milk, Milk Substitutes, & Milk Products   62

Noodles & Pasta, Plain   64

Nuts & Nut-based Butters, Flours, Meals, Milks,
    Pastes, & Powders   64

Pickles & Relishes   70

Pizza   70

Pork, Fresh & Cured   71

Poultry, Fresh & Processed   71

Processed Meat & Poultry Products   73

Rice & Grains, Plain & Prepared   73

Salad Dressings & Mayonnaise   75

Sauces & Gravies   76

Seafood & Seafood Products   77

Seasonings   78

Seeds & Seed-based Butters, Flours, & Meals   80

Snacks   82

Soups, Prepared   83

Soybeans & Soybean Products   88

Sugars & Sweeteners   90

Vegetables, Plain & Prepared   90

Acknowledgments

I would like to thank Leah Wallach, who paved the way with the first three books in this series and provided much-needed advice and information for this one. I also want to thank the consumer-affairs people at the many food manufacturers who provided information for brand-name products; Jean Stewart of the United States Department of Agriculture for her help with generic foods; Dr. Kelly Long of Rice University in Houston and Dr. William Henrich of the Southwestern Medical School in Dallas for their advice on the introductory material; Carol Hornig, nutritionist; and my husband for his help throughout. Kudos also to my agent, Joe Spieler, who helped with all the mail, and Carol Cohen and Eric Wirth at Harper & Row.

Introduction

Oat bran, a common fiber, is officially classified as a non-nutritive substance. It has been an ingredient in many breakfast cereals, but we now find oat bran boldly advertised as a valuable ingredient in everything from brownies to potato chips. Why is this "non-nutritive substance" suddenly deemed so important in our diet?

The answer takes us all the way back to 1840, when an American doctor determined that "coarse brown bread" was beneficial in the treatment of constipation. We then move up to the period following World War II, when two doctors working in the central African kingdom of Uganda realized that the rural villagers were amazingly free of certain diseases of the colon common in Western countries. The "fiber hypothesis" was born. Studies of eating habits around the world multiplied in the 1970s and 1980s, and what had initially been a mere hypothesis was shown to be a "fiber fact": the consumption of unrefined, high-fiber carbohydrate foods—a typical diet in many underdeveloped countries—has the beneficial effect of reducing the incidence of colon cancer, diverticular disease of the colon, and diabetes and can also help alleviate constipation and other problems of the digestive system.

Most nutritionists now acknowledge the value of greater quantities of fiber in the typical Western diet. Thus the boom in oat bran.

What Is Fiber?

Fiber is the term that denotes the tough, fibrous parts of plant cell walls and some compounds found inside those walls—that portion of cereals, fruits, beans, vegetables, nuts, and seeds that cannot be broken down by the enzymes of the gastrointestinal tract and thus reaches the colon undigested. Fiber used to be called "roughage" or "unavailable carbohydrates." These terms were replaced by "crude fiber," a measurement that is outdated but still in use and will therefore be explained later. The new standard term and measuring stick is *dietary* fiber.

Components and Functions of Dietary Fiber

Dietary fiber has many components, and each component has a special function in the body. The major impact of dietary fiber is in the colon, the last part of the gastrointestinal tract, but the addition of fibrous foods to the diet increases the bulk of the food all along the tract. Many health experts believe that fiber exercises the muscles of the digestive tract, speeds up the flow of food through the digestive tract, modulates the size and consistency of the stool, binds certain lipids and carries them out of the body, binds and reduces the absorption of salts in the intestinal tract, and modulates the body's response to glucose.

For the layperson interested in nutrition, the most important distinction between the fiber components and their functions in the body is that some fibers are *insoluble* in water and some are *water-soluble*, and their effects on the digestive system vary accordingly. Insoluble fibers act like a sponge, soaking up water in the digestive tract. Water-soluble fibers generally act as a laxative by forming a gel with water. Consumption of both types of fiber is necessary in order to receive all the possible benefits.

Insoluble Fiber   Insoluble dietary fibers, which are found in fruits, vegetables, beans, and oats, include cellulose, lignin, and hemicellulose. Cellulose is the main component of plant cell walls. It is resistant to salivary and pancreatic amylase, but it is capable of being broken down by the cellulases of the colonic bacteria. Lignin is the noncarbohydrate component in the fiber category. It is an inert, woody substance that is even more resistant to digestion than other fibers and acts like a structural binding agent.

Hemicellulose is partially water-soluble, but it has a similar effect on the digestive tract as cellulose. It has a good water-holding capacity, digestibility, and capacity to bind trace minerals, salts, and bile acids.

The specific effects of insoluble fibers are many. Functioning as a sponge, they increase the bulk of the wastes in the digestive tract, adding mass to the stool and making it easier to pass. Some researchers believe that this action may also dilute cancer-causing substances while helping to remove them from the digestive system. Cellulose appears to reduce glucose levels in the blood, and lignin is thought to be especially productive in easing the removal of cholesterol and acids from the intestinal tract. It may also protect against the formation of gallstones. Insoluble fibers may also benefit people on diets. The fact that these unabsorbed fibers literally take up space in the digestive system makes us feel full more quickly and maintain that feeling for longer periods of time.

Water-Soluble Fiber   Water-soluble dietary fibers, which are found in wheat, corn bran, and cereal grains, include gums, mucilages, and pectin. These fibers act as a laxative by forming a gel with water, prolonging the transit time of materials through the intestine (offsetting the effects of the insoluble fibers, which tend to decrease that time). It is suggested that the gels of water-soluble fibers also trap sugar and bind cholesterol, thereby slowing the absorption of these compounds into the bloodstream. Health-care specialists are also discovering that these fibers are beneficial in treating diabetes, because they reduce the body's insulin requirements.

Gums are the sticky excretions from the plant walls and are essentially nondigestible by us. Research suggests that gums coat the lining of the stomach, slowing down the absorption of whatever we have eaten, and they can lower cholesterol levels significantly. Mucilages are the secretions of plant seeds that prevent dehydration. They are very hard to digest. Pectin, known by jam and jelly makers for its ability to form gels, aids absorption in the stomach and the bowels and may be effective countering cholesterol.

Fiber and Your Health

Research on the various benefits of fiber is still in its infancy, but credible research is leading physicians to consider increased-fiber diets in the treatment of these medical problems:

- *Constipation*: The ability of insoluble fiber to hold water enables the contents of the bowels to remain large and soft. A lack of fiber results in water loss, which causes stools to be firm yet small. Therefore, with more water in the digestive tract, there will be better elimination.

- *Diverticulosis*: Diverticulosis is believed to be caused by pressure on the intestinal walls from the passage of hard, dry stools or from chronic constipation. The softening and bulking of the stool due to the presence of fiber eases elimination and lowers the necessary muscular pressure.

- *Irritable bowel syndrome*: A diet rich in fiber can help release gas pockets with its laxative effect. Severe abdominal gas and pain, usually accompanied by constipation and diarrhea in irritable bowel syndrome, is relieved.

- *Colon cancer*: A diet rich in fiber may help clear the body of toxins that can accumulate in the colon and result in cancer.

- *High cholesterol*: Fiber, especially lignin and pectin, may reduce serum cholesterol.

- *Diabetes*: Studies indicate that the glucose and endocrine responses to "test meals" may be reduced by the addition of fiber to the diet.

- *Gallstones*: Fiber is thought to bind cholesterol and bile acids to the stool. It also promotes the production of chenodeoxycholate, a substance that helps dissolve gallstones.

- *Hemorrhoids and hiatus hernia*: Hemorrhoids and hiatus hernia may be the result of increased abdominal pressure in attempts to pass constipated stools. Fiber is considered to deter these conditions, since it regulates the bowels and softens stools, preventing increased abdominal pressure.

• *Weight control*: Foods high in fiber tend to be low in fat
and simple sugars. Also, high-fiber foods, because of their
water-holding capacity, satisfy hunger readily.

How Much and What Kind of Fiber Do We Need?

Currently there is no recommended daily allowance for dietary fiber. The estimated level of total dietary fiber intake in the typical Western diet is less than 20 grams per day. Those eating a moderately high-fiber diet probably consume around 35 grams per day and those on a strict vegetarian diet around 60 grams a day. The National Cancer Institute has suggested that Americans try to eat between 25 and 35 grams per day. Some doctors and nutritionists estimate the average American should consume at least 60 grams of dietary fiber a day. Yet consumption of certain high-fiber diets has been associated with zinc deficiency, sigmoid volvulus, and esophageal cancer. The jury is still out.

While trying to increase our consumption of fiber, the caloric "side effects" of high-fiber foods should be taken into account. Nuts are rich in fiber but are also high in calories. On a fiber/calorie basis the leafy green vegetables are good sources, as are certain root vegetables, such as parsnips and carrots.

As noted earlier, insoluble fibers are found mainly in fruits, vegetables, beans, and oats. Water-soluble fibers are found predominantly in wheat, corn bran, and cereal grains. Some foods are composed of both soluble and insoluble fibers. Bran and whole-grain cereals contain cellulose (insoluble), hemicellulose (insoluble), and pectin (soluble). Carrots, sweet corn, peas, potatoes, pears, raspberries, and strawberries have high concentrations of cellulose (insoluble), pectin (soluble), and lignin (insoluble).

Fiber Labeling

Fiber is reported on nutritional labels and other food-value tables as either crude or dietary. *Crude* fiber is the term most of us are familiar with. It is the term found on the nutritional labels of most packaged foods, if fiber is listed at all. (Listing of fiber is not required by the FDA.) Crude fiber has been measured since the last century by sequentially digesting a food sample with acids and bases. Whatever is left is the measurement of crude fiber. But when humans eat the same food, subjecting it to their own digestive enzymes, the undigested portion will be greater than the laboratory portion because human digestive juices are less harsh than the laboratory acids and bases. The more useful measurement is how much fiber remains in the body after the normal human digestive process. This is called *dietary* fiber. Crude fiber is therefore an outdated concept.

Testing for dietary fiber is becoming more common, and nutritional data and product labeling are increasingly indicating dietary rather than crude fiber. Until the dietary fiber measurement is standard, however, the rule of thumb to use for the relationship between crude and dietary is that for every gram of crude fiber in a given food, there are probably two or three grams of dietary fiber.

Although dietary fiber is a more complete picture of the amount of fiber we have consumed for our bodies to use, some feel that this measurement is still not helpful enough because of the diversity of the effects of fiber. One researcher has concluded that the simple label *dietary fiber* is "no more helpful than one that states vitamin content without specifying the vitamins." Nevertheless, the product labeling on the market today provides no distinctions among the dietary fibers.

How to Use This Book

Food Values: Fiber provides the number of grams of fiber and the total number of calories in thousands of foods.

The foods are divided into forty-five categories covering all the things we eat and drink. As you flip through the pages of this book you'll quickly see where various foods are located. If you can't find a food in the category where you think it belongs, check the head note at the beginning of the category or refer to the table of contents. When products could be classified in more than one category, we have tried to include a "see also" reference.

Each category begins with an alphabetical listing of generic food items, with fresh products listed before processed foods: for instance, you'll find fresh peaches before canned peaches. Following the generic foods are all brand-name products alphabetized by the name that is most easily recognized—the name of the manufacturing company, of the product line, or of the product itself. For instance, General Mills cereals are listed under General Mills, the company name, while Erewhon cereals are listed under Erewhon, the product line, rather than the manufacturer, U.S. Mills. Under each brand name, specific products are generally listed alphabetically: Aunt Jemima French toast, for example, precedes Aunt Jemima pancakes. We found, however, as most alphabetizers do, that some items could be listed in more than one way; we had to make choices. Thousand Island low-calorie dressing follows Thousand Island regular dressing, for example, and split peas are under *s*, not *p*. If you don't find a food under the first letter of the first word of its name, try looking for it under the first letter of another word in the name. The cross-references should help here too.

Be sure to look for foods in the form in which you eat them: the way foods are prepared changes their nutrient values. An apple, applesauce, and apple juice contain different amounts of fiber.

We've used the portion sizes that Americans use—cups, ounces, or serving units—and when they're available, we've used two kinds of measures; for example, "3 cookies = 1 oz." Serving units are the easiest portions to measure: it's easier to count cookies than to weigh them. However, you can compare only serving units of the same weight. If a package of Brand X frozen lasagna weighs 10 ounces and a package of Brand Y frozen lasagna weighs 18 ounces, Brand Y will probably contain more calories and fiber, because the portion size is larger. But Brand Y might contain fewer calories and less fiber per ounce. To compare two products of different sizes, divide the values for each product by the number of ounces they contain, and then compare the values for 1 ounce.

Also note the difference between weight measures and volume measures. Measuring cups measure fluid ounces. An ounce of water by weight fills a measuring cup to the 1-ounce line. But volume and weight are very different kinds of measures for solid foods. An ounce of unpopped popcorn, which is dense, wouldn't fill a measuring cup, for example, but an ounce of popped popcorn, which is airy, would fill more than one. In this book, portions for solid food given in ounces refer to weight. Fluid ounces (fl oz), cups (c), teaspoons (t), and tablespoons (T) refer to volume measurements. Since we don't ordinarily weigh our food, volume and weight measurements are given when both are available and useful. For example, we've indicated how much of a measuring cup would be filled by an ounce of a given cold cereal when this information is available.

All values given here are approximations. No two apples, chicken breasts, or rolls are exactly alike. Data represent averages for several samples.

Figures provided by different sources may not be exactly comparable. The U.S. Department of Agriculture (USDA) and various manufacturers often use different analytical procedures to analyze nutrient content and may round off the data in different ways. In the USDA *Composition of Food* series, our source of information about generic and fresh food, values are given to hundredths and thousandths. Figures for fiber are given in *Food Values: Fiber* in the form in which they were provided by the source of nutrient information. If a fiber figure is followed by the symbol • it refers to crude fiber; otherwise, the figure refers to dietary fiber.

We rounded off calorie figures, however, to the nearest whole unit. For example, we list 68.4 calories as 68 calories and 68.5 calories as 69 calories. When an item contained less than .5 calories we listed the value as a "trace" (tr). Many manufacturers use a simpler rounding-off system for calories, approved by the Food and Drug Administration, which regulates food labels. Calories between 0 and 20 may be given in increments of 2; between 20 and 50 in increments of 5; and above 50 in increments of 5 or 10. This means that there's no point in counting single calories when comparing products; a product listed as containing 197 calories, another as 195 calories, and a third as 200 calories may actually contain the same amount of food energy. For most practical purposes, these small differences don't matter. If you need about 2,000 calories a day, it doesn't matter if you get 2,005 one day and 1,991 the next.

This book contains the best and most complete information now available. Since food manufacturers constantly change recipes and product sizes and develop new products, some of the data contained here may quickly become outdated.

Calculating the Number of Grams of Fiber in Your Diet

To get an idea of how many grams of fiber are in your present diet, keep a record of everything you eat and drink for three days, preferably including one weekend day. Right after you finish a meal, snack, or beverage, write down what you ate; how it was prepared; the portion by volume (cups, tablespoons), weight (ounces, pounds), or units (one medium apple, one English muffin); or all three if you can. To get a feeling for different food sizes, measure your food when you are at home. For example, instead of just pouring cereal from the box into a bowl, weigh or measure it first to see how much you use. Use tablespoons to measure the wheat germ you put into your yogurt. You may find that the portion sizes used in the book are smaller than the ones you use.

At the end of three days, look up the fiber and calorie values for every food on your list. Add them up and divide by three to get your average daily intake. We have given the dietary fiber amount when available, but much of the data still reflects only the crude fiber (those figures followed by • in the book). Therefore, you will have to add up all the crude and dietary values separately. Multiply the crude figure by two or three to obtain the estimated dietary equivalent. Then add the two totals to determine average daily intake.

Sources

1. *Food Values of Portions Commonly Used, 14th Edition*, Jean A. T. Pennington and Helen Nichols Church, Harper & Row, 1985.
2. *Nutritive Value of Foods*, U.S. Department of Agriculture, Nutrition Information Service, Home and Garden Bulletin #72, revised 1981.
3. *Composition of Food Series*, U.S. Department of Agriculture, Science and Education Administration:

   8-1 *Dairy and Egg Products*, revised November 1976.
   8-3 *Baby Foods*, revised December 1978.
   8-4 *Fats and Oils*, revised June 1979.
   8-5 *Poultry Products*, revised August 1979.
   8-6 *Soups, Sauces and Gravies*, revised February 1980.
   8-7 *Sausages and Luncheon Meats*, revised September 1980.
   8-8 *Breakfast Cereals*, revised July 1982.
   8-9 *Fruits and Fruit Juices*, revised August 1982.
   8-10 *Pork Products*, revised August 1983.
   8-11 *Vegetables and Vegetable Products*, revised August 1984.
   8-12 *Nut and Seed Products*, revised September 1984.
   8-13 *Beef Products*, revised August 1986.
   8-14 *Beverages*, revised May 1986.
   8-15 *Finfish and Shellfish Products*, revised September 1987.
   8-16 *Legumes and Legume Products*, revised December 1986.

Information about brand-name products was supplied by the food processing companies themselves or taken from the above sources.

Abbreviations

c	=	cup
diam	=	diameter
g	=	grams
lb	=	pounds
mg	=	milligrams
oz	=	ounces
pkg	=	package
pkt	=	packet
T	=	tablespoon
t	=	teaspoon
tr	=	trace
w/	=	with
w/out	=	without

	Portion	Fiber (g)	Calories

❏ BABY FOOD *See* INFANT & TODDLER FOODS

❏ BAKING INGREDIENTS

	Portion	Fiber (g)	Calories
candied fruit			
apricot	1 medium	0.2 •	101
cherry	3 large	0.1 •	51
citron	1 oz	0.4 •	89
fig	1 piece	1.3 •	90
ginger root	1 oz	0.2 •	95
maraschino cherry	2 medium	0.1 •	19
pear	1 oz	0.3 •	85
peel of grapefruit/lemon/ orange	1 oz	0.6 •	89
pineapple	1 slice	0.3 •	120
cornmeal *See* FLOURS & CORNMEALS			
cornstarch *See* FLOURS & CORNMEALS			
flour *See* FLOURS & CORNMEALS			
piecrust			
crumb	5.8 oz	0.3 •	866
graham cracker	4.8 oz	0.2 •	159
yeast			
torula	1 T	0.3 •	28

❏ BAKING MIXES

cakes & pastries, prepared from mix *See* DESSERTS: CAKES, PASTRIES, & PIES
pancakes, prepared from mix *See* BREAKFAST FOODS, PREPARED
waffles, prepared from mix *See* BREAKFAST FOODS, PREPARED

Fiber figures marked with • refer to *crude* fiber. Unmarked fiber figures refer to *dietary* fiber.

	Portion	Fiber (g)	Calories

■ **BRAND NAME**

Aunt Jemima
Easy Mix coffee cake	1.3 oz	0.7	156
Easy Mix corn bread	1.7 oz	1.4	196

Fearn
bran muffin mix	1½ oz	8	110
carob cake mix	⅓ c dry	6	120
whole-wheat baking mix	½ c	9	210

Flako
corn muffin mix	1 oz	0.7	116
pie crust mix	1.7 oz	1.2	247

❑ **BEANS** *See* LEGUMES & LEGUME PRODUCTS

❑ **BEEF, FRESH & CURED**

Fresh & cured beef & beef variety meats contain no dietary fiber.

❑ **BEVERAGES**

Carbonated Beverages

Carbonated beverages contain no dietary fiber.

Coffee & Coffee Substitutes

coffee substitute, cereal grain beverage, powder			
prepared w/water	6 fl oz water + 1 t powder	0.0 •	9
prepared w/whole milk	6 fl oz milk + 1 t powder	0.0 •	121

	Portion	Fiber (g)	Calories
Flavored Milk Beverages			
carob-flavored mix			
powder	3 t	0.2 •	45
powder, prepared w/whole milk	1 c milk + 3 t powder	0.2 •	195
chocolate-flavored mix			
powder	2–3 heaping t	0.2 •	75
powder, prepared w/whole milk	1 c milk + 2–3 heaping t powder	0.2 •	226
chocolate milk			
whole	1 c	0.15 •	208
low-fat, 2%	1 c	0.15 •	179
low-fat, 1%	1 c	0.15 •	158
chocolate syrup			
w/added nutrients	1 T	0.1 •	46
prepared w/whole milk	1 c milk + 1 T syrup	0.1 •	196
w/out added nutrients	1 fl oz	0.1 •	82
prepared w/whole milk	1 c milk + 2 T syrup	0.1 •	232
cocoa mix, w/out added nutrients	6 fl oz water + 3–4 heaping t powder	0.2 •	103
cocoa, homemade, w/whole milk	6 fl oz	0.15 •	164
	1 c	0.20 •	218
eggnog, dairy	1 c	0 •	342
eggnog-flavored mix, powder, prepared w/whole milk	1 c milk + 2 heaping t powder	0.0 •	260
malted milk–flavored mix, chocolate			
w/added nutrients			
powder	¾ oz or 4–5 heaping t	0.0 •	75
powder, prepared w/whole milk	1 c milk + 4–5 heaping t powder	0.0 •	225

Fiber figures marked with • refer to *crude* fiber. Unmarked fiber figures refer to *dietary* fiber.

	Portion	Fiber (g)	Calories
malted milk–flavored mix, chocolate *(cont.)*			
w/out added nutrients			
powder	¾ oz or 3 heaping t	0.0 •	79
powder, prepared w/whole milk	1 c milk + 3 heaping t powder	0.0 •	229
malted milk–flavored mix, natural			
w/added nutrients			
powder	¾ oz or 4–5 heaping t	0.0 •	80
powder, prepared w/whole milk	1 c milk + 4–5 heaping t powder	0.0 •	230
w/out added nutrients			
powder	¾ oz or 3 heaping t	0.0 •	87
powder, prepared w/whole milk	1 c milk + 3 heaping t powder	0.0 •	237
shake, thick			
chocolate	10.6 oz	0.75 •	356
vanilla	about 11 oz	0.19 •	350

Fruit & Vegetable Juices

	Portion	Fiber (g)	Calories
acerola	1 c	0.73 •	51
apple, canned or bottled	1 c	0.52 •	116
apricot, canned	1 c	0.48 •	141
carrot, canned	½ c	1.17 •	49
lemon, frozen, single strength	1 T	0.05 •	3
orange			
fresh	1 c	0.25 •	111
canned	1 c	0.25 •	104
from frozen concentrate	1 c	0.13 •	112
frozen concentrate, undiluted	6 fl oz	0.39 •	339
passion fruit			
purple	1 c	0.10 •	126
yellow	1 c	0.42 •	149
peach, canned	1 c	0.35 •	134
pear, canned	1 c	0.78 •	149
pineapple			
canned	1 c	0.25 •	139
from frozen concentrate	1 c	0.25 •	129

	Portion	Fiber (g)	Calories
prune, canned	1 c	0.03 •	181
tangerine			
fresh	1 c	0.25 •	106
canned, sweetened	1 c	0.25 •	125
tomato, canned	6 fl oz	0.72 •	32
w/beef broth	5½ fl oz	0.2 •	61
vegetable, canned	6 fl oz	0.42 •	34

Fruit Juice Drinks (10–50% Fruit Juice), Juice Ades, & Juice-flavored Drinks & Powders

apple juice drink, canned	6 fl oz	tr •	92
cherry juice drink, canned	6 fl oz	tr •	93
citrus fruit drink, canned	6 fl oz	0.2 •	93
Florida punch juice drink, canned	6 fl oz	0.2 •	95
lemon-lime, from mix	8 fl oz	tr •	91
lemonade, from frozen concentrate	1 c	0.1 •	100
orange & apricot juice drink, canned	1 c	0.5 •	128
orange-pineapple juice drink, canned	6 fl oz	0.1 •	94
peach juice drink, canned	6 fl oz	0.1 •	90
pineapple & grapefruit juice drink, canned	1 c	0.1 •	117
pineapple-orange juice drink, canned	6 fl oz	0.0 •	99
tangerine juice drink, canned	6 fl oz	tr •	90
wild berry juice drink, canned	6 fl oz	tr •	88

Tea

instant, powder			
low-cal, sodium-saccharin-sweetened, lemon-flavored	2 t	0 •	5
sugar-sweetened, lemon-flavored	3 rounded t	0 •	87
unsweetened	1 t	0 •	2
unsweetened, lemon-flavored	1 rounded t	0 •	4

Fiber figures marked with • refer to *crude* fiber. Unmarked fiber figures refer to *dietary* fiber.

	Portion	Fiber (g)	Calories
Water			
municipal	1 c	0 •	0

▪ BRAND NAME

Awake			
from frozen concentrate	6 fl oz	0.1 •	91
Orange Plus			
from frozen concentrate	6 fl oz	0.1 •	97

❏ BREADCRUMBS, CROUTONS, STUFFINGS, & SEASONED COATINGS

cornflake crumbs	1 oz	tr •	110
croutons, herb-seasoned	0.7 oz	0.2 •	70
stuffing, corn bread, from mix	½ c	0.3 •	117

▪ BRAND NAME

Arnold Croutons			
Cheddar Romano Crispy	½ oz	0.3	64
Cheese Garlic Crispy	½ oz	0.4	60
Fine Herbs Crispy	½ oz	0.4	53
Italian Crispy	½ oz	0.5	62
Seasoned Crispy	½ oz	0.5	60
Devonsheer Breadcrumbs			
plain	1 oz	0.9	108
Italian Style	1 oz	0.9	104

❏ BREADS, ROLLS, BISCUITS, & MUFFINS

Bread & Bread Sticks

bread sticks			
regular	1	tr •	23
Vienna	1	tr •	18

	Portion	Fiber (g)	Calories
corn bread			
from mix	1 piece	1.7 •	178
homemade			
w/enriched cornmeal	2.9 oz	0.1 •	198
w/whole-ground cornmeal	2.7 oz	0.2 •	172
honey wheatberry bread	1 oz slice	0.1 •	70
sourdough bread	1 oz slice	0.1 •	68
wheatberry bread	1 oz slice	0.4 •	70

Muffins

English, sourdough	2 oz	0.2 •	129

Rolls & Bagels

brown & serve roll	1	tr •	92
parkerhouse roll	0.6 oz	0.1 •	59
raisin roll	2.1 oz	0.5 •	165
rye roll	0.6 oz	0.1 •	55
dark, hard	1 oz	0.1 •	80
light, hard	1 oz	0.1 •	79
sandwich roll	1.8 oz	0.3 •	162
sesame seed roll	0.6 oz	0.1 •	59
wheat roll	0.6 oz	0.1 •	52
white roll, homemade	1.2 oz	0.1 •	119
whole-wheat roll, homemade	1.2 oz	0.6 •	90

▪ BRAND NAME

Arnold
BREADS

Bakery Light Golden Wheat	1 slice	2	44
Bakery Light Italian	1 slice	2	45
Bakery Light Oatmeal	1 slice	1.9	44
Bran'nola County Oat	1 slice	2.8	90
Bran'nola Dark Wheat	1 slice	2.8	83
Bran'nola Hearty Wheat	1 slice	2.7	88
Bran'nola Nutty Grains	1 slice	3	85
Bran'nola Original	1 slice	2.9	85
Brick Oven Extra Fiber White	1 slice	2.1	55

Fiber figures marked with • refer to *crude* fiber. Unmarked fiber figures refer to *dietary* fiber.

	Portion	Fiber (g)	Calories
Brick Oven White	1 slice	0.9	79
Brown Natural Wheat	1 slice	2.3	80
cinnamon raisin	1 slice	0.8	67
Country White	1 slice	1	98
dill rye	1 slice	1.3	71
Francisco International Italian Thick Sliced	1 slice	0.9	66
honey wheatberry	1 slice	2.4	77
Jewish rye			
w/out seeds	1 slice	1.2	71
w/seeds	1 slice	1.3	70
melba thin rye	1 slice	0.9	44
#1 Brick Oven Wheat	1 slice	1.7	60
orange raisin	1 slice	0.8	67
pumpernickel	1 slice	1.3	70
stoneground 100% whole wheat	1 slice	1.6	48

ROLLS

	Portion	Fiber (g)	Calories
Dinner Party roll	1	0.8	51
Dutch egg sandwich bun	1	1.9	123
hamburger bun	1	1.8	115
soft sandwich roll	1	1.7	110
Lender's Bagels			
onion	1	0.12 •	160
pumpernickel	1	0.3 •	160
Wheat 'n Raisin	1	0.64 •	190
Levy's Jewish Rye			
w/out seeds	1 slice	1.3	75
w/seeds	1 slice	1.4	76
Sahara Pita Bread			
wheat	1 miniloaf	2.4	66
Thomas's Breads			
Fiber Calcium	1 slice	2.7	52
Lite Wheat	1 slice	2.1	41

❑ BREAKFAST CEREALS, COLD & HOT

Cold Cereal

	Portion	Fiber (g)	Calories
cornflakes, low-sodium	1 oz or about 1 c	0.2 •	113

	Portion	Fiber (g)	Calories
crisp rice			
regular	1 oz or about 1 c	0.4	112
low-sodium	1 oz or about 1 c	0.1 •	114
granola, homemade	1 oz or about ¼ c	0.4 •	138
	1 c	1.7 •	595
honey bran	1 oz or about ⅞ c	3.1	97
	1 c	3.9	119
oat flakes, fortified	1 oz or about ⅔ c	0.7	105
	1 c	1.2	177
raisins, rice & rye	1.3 oz or about 1 c	0.4 •	124
rice, puffed	½ oz or about 1 c	0.1	57
sugar-sparkled flakes	1 oz box	0.1 •	109
wheat, puffed, plain	½ oz or about 1 c (heaping)	0.5	52
wheat, shredded			
large biscuit	1 rectangular	2.2	83
	2 round	3.5	133
small biscuit	1 oz or about ⅔ c	2.6	102
	⅞ oz box	2.3	89
wheat germ, toasted			
plain	1 oz or about ¼ c	0.7 •	108
	1 c	2.6 •	431
w/brown sugar & honey	1 oz or about ¼ c	0.5 •	107
	1 c	1.9 •	426

Hot Cereal

	Portion	Fiber (g)	Calories
corn grits			
regular & quick			
dry	1 c	2.5	579
	1 T	0.2	36

Fiber figures marked with • refer to *crude* fiber. Unmarked fiber figures refer to *dietary* fiber.

	Portion	Fiber (g)	Calories
corn grits: regular & quick *(cont.)*			
cooked	1 c	0.6	146
	¾ c	0.5	110
instant, prepared			
plain	1 pkt	0.1 •	82
w/artificial cheese flavor	1 pkt	0.2 •	107
w/imitation bacon bits	1 pkt	0.2 •	104
w/imitation ham bits	1 pkt	0.2 •	103
farina			
dry	1 c	0.3 •	649
	1 T	0.0 •	40
cooked	1 c	0.1 •	116
	¾ c	0.1 •	87
grits; hominy grits *See* corn grits, *above*			
oats, regular, quick, & instant, nonfortified			
dry	⅓ c	1.5	104
cooked	1 c	2.1	145
	¾ c	1.6	108

• BRAND NAME

Arrowhead Mills
COLD CEREAL

Agrain & Agrain	2 oz	6.9	220
Arrowhead Crunch	1 oz	3.46	120
bran flakes	1 oz	4.06	100
corn, puffed	½ oz	0.49	50
cornflakes	1 oz	2.78	110
granola			
apple amaranth	2 oz	6.75	225
maple nut	2 oz	7.85	260
millet, puffed	½ oz	0.49	50
Nature O's	1 oz	2.84	110
rice, puffed	½ oz	0.41	50
wheat, puffed	½ oz	0.86	50
wheat bran	2 oz	24.48	200
wheat germ, raw	2 oz	6.47	210

HOT CEREAL

Bear Mush	1 oz	1.33	100
corn grits, yellow	2 oz	1.47	200
4 Grain & Flax	2 oz	7.32	94

	Portion	Fiber (g)	Calories
oat bran	1 oz	6.24	110
oatmeal, instant	1 oz	4.20	100
Seven Grain	1 oz	3.89	100

Erewhon
COLD CEREAL

	Portion	Fiber (g)	Calories
Crispy Brown Rice			
regular	1 oz or about 1 c	4	110
low-sodium	1 oz or about 1 c	4	110
#9 granola, w/bran, no salt added	1 oz or about ¼ c	4	130
raisin bran	1 oz or about ½ c	3	100
wheat flakes	1 oz or about ½ c	3.5	110

HOT CEREAL

	Portion	Fiber (g)	Calories
oat bran w/toasted wheat germ	1 oz or about ⅓ c dry	3	115

General Mills Cold Cereal

	Portion	Fiber (g)	Calories
Cheerios			
regular	1 oz or about 1¼ c	1.1	111
	¾ oz box	0.8	83
Honey Nut	1 oz or about ¾ c	0.3 •	107
	1 c	0.4 •	125
Crispy Wheats 'n Raisins	1 oz or about ¾ c	1.3	99
	1 c	2.0	150
Golden Grahams	1 oz or about ¾ c	0.5	109
	1 c	0.7	150
Kix	1 oz or about 1½ c	0.4	110
	¾ oz box	0.3	83
Lucky Charms	1 oz or about 1 c	0.6	110

Fiber figures marked with • refer to *crude* fiber. Unmarked fiber figures refer to *dietary* fiber.

	Portion	Fiber (g)	Calories
Total	1 oz or about 1 c	2.0	100
Trix	1 oz or about 1 c	0.1	109
Wheaties	1 oz or about 1 c	2.0	99

Health Valley
COLD CEREAL

	Portion	Fiber (g)	Calories
Amaranth Crunch w/raisins	1 oz or about ¼ c	2.7	120
amaranth flakes	1 oz or about ½ c	2.8	110
amaranth w/banana	1 oz or about ¼ c	4.2	114
bran			
w/apples & cinnamon	1 oz or about ¼ c	5.1	110
w/raisins	1 oz or about ¼ c	4.5	108
Fiber 7 Flakes	1 oz or about ½ c	3.6	113
Fruit Lites			
corn	½ oz or about ½ c	0.12	48
rice	½ oz or about ½ c	0.11	48
wheat	½ oz or about ½ c	0.61	48
granola *See* Real Granola, *below*			
Healthy Crunch			
w/almonds & dates	1 oz or about ¼ c	1.6	120
w/apples & cinnamon	1 oz or about ¼ c	1.6	120
oat bran flakes			
plain	1 oz or about ½ c	2.8	117
w/almonds & dates	1 oz or about ½ c	2.8	105
w/raisins	1 oz or about ½ c	2.8	105
Orangeola			
w/almonds & dates	1 oz or about ¼ c	3.6	120

	Portion	Fiber (g)	Calories
w/banana & Hawaiian fruit	1 oz or about ¼ c	3.6	128
raisin bran flakes	1 oz or about ½ c	3.8	108
Real Granola			
w/almond crunch or w/Hawaiian fruit	1 oz or about ¼ c	3.6	123
w/raisins & nuts	1 oz or about ¼ c	2.49	120
Sprouts 7			
w/bananas & Hawaiian fruit	1 oz or about ¼ c	4.3	90
w/raisins	1 oz or about ¼ c	4.7	105
stoned-wheat flakes	1 oz or about ½ c	3.8	108
Swiss Breakfast			
raisin nut	1 oz or about ¼ c	3	120
tropical fruit	1 oz or about ¼ c	3	120
wheat bran/Millers Flakes	1 oz or about ½ c	11.7	118
wheat germ w/fiber, almonds & dates	1 oz or about ¼ c	4.7	92
wheat germ w/fiber, bananas & tropical fruit	1 oz or about ¼ c	4.7	100
HOT CEREAL			
hot oat bran w/apples	1 oz or about ¼ c	3.8	100
Heartland Cold Cereal			
Natural Cereal			
plain	1 oz or about ¼ c	1.3	123
	1 c	5.4	499
w/coconut	1 oz or about ¼ c	1.4	125
	1 c	5	463

Fiber figures marked with • refer to *crude* fiber. Unmarked fiber figures refer to *dietary* fiber.

	Portion	Fiber (g)	Calories
Natural Cereal *(cont.)*			
w/raisins	1 oz or about ¼ c	1.3	120
	1 c	5.1	467
Kellogg's Cold Cereal			
All-Bran	1 oz or about ⅓ c	10	70
w/extra fiber	1 oz or about ½ c	13	60
w/fruit & almonds	1.3 oz or about ⅔ c	11	100
Apple Jacks	1 oz or about 1 c	1	110
Bran Buds	1 oz or about ⅓ c	10	70
bran flakes	1 oz or about ⅔ c	5	90
Corn Flakes			
regular	1 oz or about 1 c	1	110
honey & nut	1 oz or about ⅔ c	tr	110
Corn Pops	1 oz or about 1 c	tr	110
Cracklin' Oat Bran	1 oz or about ½ c	5	110
Crispix	1 oz or about 1 c	tr	110
Froot Loops	1 oz or about 1 c	1	110
Frosted Mini-Wheats	1 oz = about 4 biscuits	3	100
Fruitful Bran	1.3 oz or about ⅔ c	5	110
Honey Smacks	1 oz or about ¾ c	1	110
Just Right			
Fruit, Nut, & Flake	1.3 oz or about ¾ c	2	140
Nugget & Flake	1 oz or about ⅔ c	2	100
Müeslix			
bran	1 oz or about ½ c	5	130
Five Grain	1 oz or about ½ c	3	150

	Portion	Fiber (g)	Calories
Nutri-Grain			
almond raisin	1.4 oz or about ⅔ c	3	140
corn	1 oz or about ½ c	3	100
wheat	1 oz or about ⅔ c	3	100
wheat & raisins	1.4 oz or about ⅔ c	3	130
Product 19	1 oz or about 1 c	1	100
raisin bran	1.4 oz or about ¾ c	5	120
Maltex			
Maltex hot cereal	1 oz	3	105
Malt-O-Meal Hot Cereal			
Malt-O-Meal, plain or chocolate			
dry	1 T	0.1 •	38
cooked	1 c	0.2 •	122
	¾ c	0.2 •	92
Maypo			
30-Second Oatmeal	1 oz	2	100
Vermont-Style Hot Oat Cereal	1 oz	2	105
Nabisco Cold Cereal			
Fruit Wheats			
apple or strawberry	1 oz	3	100
raisin	1 oz	3	100
100% Bran	1 oz or about ½ c	10	70
Shredded Wheat 'n Bran	1 oz	4	110
Team	1 oz or about 1 c	0.3	110
Toasted Wheat & Raisins	1 oz	3	100
Nature Valley Cold Cereal			
granola, toasted oat mixture	1 oz or about ⅓ c	1.0	126
	1 c	4.2	503
Post Cold Cereal			
Alpha-Bits	1 oz	1	110

Fiber figures marked with • refer to *crude* fiber. Unmarked fiber figures refer to *dietary* fiber.

	Portion	Fiber (g)	Calories
C.W. Post Hearty Granola			
plain	1 oz	1	130
w/raisins	1 oz	1	120
Cocoa Pebbles	1 oz	tr	110
Fruit & Fibre: dates, raisins, walnuts; Harvest Medley; Mountain Trail; or tropical fruit	1 oz	4	90
Fruity Pebbles	1 oz	tr	110
granola *See* C.W. Post Hearty Granola, *above*			
Grape-Nuts			
regular	1 oz	2	110
raisin	1 oz	2	100
Grape-Nuts Flakes	1 oz	2	100
Honeycomb	1 oz	tr	110
Natural Bran Flakes	1 oz	5	90
Natural Raisin Bran	1 oz	4	80
oat flakes, fortified	1 oz	1	110
Post Toasties	1 oz	tr	110
Super Golden Crisp	1 oz or about ⅞ c	tr	110

Quaker Oats
COLD CEREAL

	Portion	Fiber (g)	Calories
bran, unprocessed	0.25 oz	3.3	8
Cap'n Crunch			
regular	1 oz or about ¾ c	0.8	113
peanut butter	1 oz or about ¾ c	0.8	119
w/Crunchberries	1 oz or about ¾ c	0.7	113
Crunchy Bran	1 oz or about ¾ c	5.2	89
Life, plain or cinnamon	1 oz or about ⅔ c	2.5	101
Oat Squares	1 oz	2.4	105
100% Natural Cereal			
plain	1 oz or about ¼ c	7.2	127
w/apples & cinnamon	1 oz or about ¼ c	1.6	126
w/raisins & dates	1 oz or about ¼ c	1.8	123

	Portion	Fiber (g)	Calories
HOT CEREAL			
oat bran	1 oz	4.2	92
oatmeal, instant, prepared			
regular	1 oz	2.8	94
w/apples & cinnamon	1.25 oz	3.0	118
w/artificial maple & brown sugar	1.5 oz	2.8	152
w/peaches & cream	1 oz	2.3	129
w/raisins & spice	1 oz	2.8	149
w/raisins, dates, & walnuts	1 oz	2.4	141
w/strawberries & cream	1 oz	2.2	129
Quaker Oats, Quick & Old Fashioned	1 oz	2.7	99
Whole Wheat Hot Natural	1 oz	2.2	92
Ralston Purina			
COLD CEREAL			
Bran Chex	1 oz or about ⅔ c	4.6	91
	1 c	7.9	156
Cookie-Crisp	1 oz or about 1 c	0.2	114
Corn Chex	1 oz or about 1 c	0.5	111
	¾ oz box	0.4	84
cornflakes	1 oz or about 1 c	0.6	111
40% bran flakes	1 oz or about ¾ c	3.5	92
	1 c	6.0	159
raisin bran	1⅓ oz or about ¾ c	4.8	120
	1 c	7.1	178
Rice Chex	1 oz or about 1⅛ c	0.2	112
	⅞ oz box	0.1	98
sugar-frosted flakes	1 oz or about ¾ c	0.4	111
	1 c	0.5	149

Fiber figures marked with • refer to *crude* fiber. Unmarked fiber figures refer to *dietary* fiber.

	Portion	Fiber (g)	Calories
Tasteeos	1 oz or about 1¼ c	1.0	111
	1 c	0.8	94
Waffelos	1 oz or about 1 c	0.4	115
Wheat Chex	1 oz or about ⅔ c	2.1	104
	1 c	3.4	169
Wheat 'n Raisin Chex	1⅓ oz or about ¾ c	2.5	130
	1 c	3.6	185

HOT CEREAL

	Portion	Fiber (g)	Calories
Ralston			
dry	¼ c	2.9	102
cooked	1 c	4.2	134
	¾ c	3.2	100
Roman Meal Hot Cereal			
Roman Meal			
plain			
dry	⅓ c	1.0 •	100
cooked	1 c	1.5 •	147
	¾ c	2.8 •	111
w/oats			
dry	¼ c	0.6 •	85
cooked	1 c	1.1 •	169
	¾ c	0.9 •	127
Sun Country Granola			
w/almonds	1 oz	1.4	130
w/raisins	1 oz	1.8	125
w/raisins & dates	1 oz	1.8	123
U.S. Mills			
See also Erewhon, above			
Skinner's raisin bran			
regular	1 oz or about ½ c	4	110
no salt added	1 oz or about ½ c	4	100
Uncle Sam cereal	1 oz or about ½ c	7	110

	Portion	Fiber (g)	Calories
Wheatena Hot Cereal			
Wheatena			
dry	¼ c	0.6 •	125
cooked	1 oz	4	100

❑ BREAKFAST FOODS, PREPARED
See also EGGS & EGG SUBSTITUTES

pancakes, homemade			
cornmeal	1 (4″ diam)	0.1 •	68
soy	1 (4″ diam)	tr •	68

▪ BRAND NAME

Aunt Jemima
FRENCH TOAST, FROZEN

original flavor	3 oz	1.3	166
cinnamon swirl	3 oz	1.3	171
raisin	3 oz	1.3	172

PANCAKE & WAFFLE MIXES

original flavor	1.3 oz	1.4	116
buckwheat	1.3 oz	5.0	143
buttermilk	1.3 oz	1.3	122
whole-wheat	1.3 oz	3.6	161

PANCAKE BATTER, FROZEN

original flavor	3.6 oz	1.8	183
blueberry	3.6 oz	1.8	204
buttermilk	3.6 oz	1.8	180

PANCAKES, FROZEN

original flavor	3.48 oz	1.8	211
blueberry	3.48 oz	1.7	220

Fiber figures marked with • refer to *crude* fiber. Unmarked fiber figures refer to *dietary* fiber.

	Portion	Fiber (g)	Calories
WAFFLES, FROZEN			
original flavor	2	1.5	173
apple & cinnamon	2	2.0	176
blueberry	2	1.3	175
buttermilk	2	1.3	179
Health Valley			
7 Sprouted Grains buttermilk pancake & biscuit mix	1 oz	3.3	100

❑ BROWNIES *See* COOKIES, BARS, & BROWNIES

❑ BUTTER
See also NUTS & NUT-BASED BUTTERS, FLOURS, MEALS, MILKS, PASTES, & POWDERS; SEEDS & SEED-BASED BUTTERS, FLOURS, & MEALS

Butter contains no dietary fiber.

❑ CAKES *See* DESSERTS: CAKES, PASTRIES, & PIES

❑ CANDIED FRUIT *See* BAKING INGREDIENTS

❑ CANDY

	Portion	Fiber (g)	Calories
caramels			
plain or chocolate	3	0.1 •	112
plain or chocolate w/nuts	2	0.1 •	120
chocolate			
chocolate fudge center	1	0.1 •	129
chocolate fudge w/nuts center	1	0.1 •	127
coconut center	1	0.2 •	123
cream center	1	0.0 •	102
fondant center	1	tr •	115

	Portion	Fiber (g)	Calories
vanilla cream center	1	tr •	114
chocolate chips			
chocolate-flavored	¼ c	0.2 •	195
dark	1 oz	0.4 •	148
milk chocolate	¼ c	0.1 •	218
chocolate-covered almonds	1 oz	0.4 •	159
chocolate-covered Brazil nuts	1 oz	0.5 •	162
chocolate kisses	6	0.3 •	154
chocolate stars	7	0.1 •	145
English toffee	1 oz	0.1 •	193
fudge			
chocolate w/nuts	1 oz	0.1 •	119
vanilla	1 oz	0.0 •	111
vanilla w/nuts	1 oz	0.1 •	119
granola bars See COOKIES, BARS, & BROWNIES			
hard candy	6 pieces	0.0 •	108
jelly beans	10	0.0 •	66
lollipop	1 medium	0.0 •	108
malted milk balls	14	0.1 •	135
marshmallows	1 large	0.0 •	25
mints	14	0.0 •	104
sugar-coated almonds	7	0.1 •	128

- **BRAND NAME**

	Portion	Fiber (g)	Calories
Mr. Goodbar	1.27 oz	0.4 •	198
Mr. Goodbar, big block	2 oz	0.6 •	300

❏ CANNED MEATS *See* PROCESSED MEAT & POULTRY PRODUCTS

❏ CEREAL, BREAKFAST *See* BREAKFAST CEREALS, COLD & HOT

Fiber figures marked with • refer to *crude* fiber. Unmarked fiber figures refer to *dietary* fiber.

	Portion	Fiber (g)	Calories

❑ CHEESE & CHEESE FOODS

Natural & process cheeses do not contain dietary fiber, unless it is introduced in other ingredients, as indicated below.

	Portion	Fiber (g)	Calories
American pasteurized process	1″ cube	tr •	66
cheese, pimiento	1 oz	tr •	106
cottage, creamed, small curd,	4 oz	tr •	140
fruit added	1 c, not packed	tr •	279

❑ CHICKEN *See* POULTRY, FRESH & PROCESSED

❑ COATINGS, SEASONED
See BREADCRUMBS, CROUTONS, STUFFINGS, & SEASONED COATINGS

❑ COOKIES, BARS, & BROWNIES

	Portion	Fiber (g)	Calories
animal cookies	15	0.1 •	120
brownies, butterscotch	1 oz	tr •	115
chocolate cookies	1	0.1 •	93
coconut bars	1	0.1 •	109
fig bars	1	0.2 •	53
molasses cookies	1	0.9 •	137
oatmeal cookies			
from mix	2	tr •	130
homemade	1	0.1 •	62
peanut butter bars	1	0.2 •	198
peanut cookies	1	0.1 •	57
sugar cookies, homemade	1	tr •	89
vanilla cream sandwich cookies	1	tr •	69

▪ BRAND NAME

Famous Amos

	Portion	Fiber (g)	Calories
chocolate chip, no nuts, extra chips	1 oz	0.11 •	147

	Portion	Fiber (g)	Calories
chocolate chip w/macadamia nuts	1 oz	0.23 •	152
chocolate chip w/pecans	1 oz	0.14 •	151
oatmeal w/cinnamon & raisins	1 oz	0.14 •	133
Health Valley			
fruit bars			
apple	2	3.10	165
date	2	2.42	180
raisin	2	2.51	160
Fruit Jumbos			
almonds & dates	1	1.11	75
oat bran	1	1.5	70
raisins & nuts	1	0.9	75
tropical fruit	1	0.9	80
graham crackers			
amaranth	7	3.11	110
oat bran	7	3.08	120
Jumbos			
amaranth	1	2.3	83
cinnamon	1	1.9	70
peanut butter	1	0.88	70
tofu cookies	4	2.9	145
wheat-free cookies	4	3.63	180
Kellogg's Rice Krispies Bars			
chocolate chip	1	0.6	120
Cocoa Krispies chocolate chip	1	0.1	120
peanut butter	1	0.2	130
Quaker Oats			
CHEWY GRANOLA BARS			
chocolate chip	1	1.4	128
chocolate, graham, & marsh-mallow	1	1.1	126
chunky nut & raisin	1	1.6	131
honey & oats	1	1.3	125
peanut butter	1	1.2	128
raisin & cinnamon	1	1.2	128

Fiber figures marked with • refer to *crude* fiber. Unmarked fiber figures refer to *dietary* fiber.

	Portion	Fiber (g)	Calories
GRANOLA DIPPS BARS			
caramel nut	1	0.7	148
chocolate chip	1	1.0	139
peanut butter	1	1	170
peanut butter & chocolate chip	1	0.2 •	174

❑ **CORNMEAL** *See* FLOURS & CORNMEALS

❑ **CRACKERS**
See also SNACKS

bread sticks *See* BREADS, ROLLS, BISCUITS, & MUFFINS			
graham *See* COOKIES, BARS, & BROWNIES			
rye crisp	¼ large square	2.5 •	40
soda, unsalted tops	10	0 •	120
zwieback *See* INFANT & TODDLER FOODS			

▪ **BRAND NAME**

Health Valley
7-Grain Vegetable			
regular	13	2.75	130
no salt	13	2.75	125
Cheese Wheels	13	2.72	150
herb, regular or no salt	13	3.46	135
honey graham	13	2.40	120
sesame, regular or no salt	13	2.55	130
stoned-wheat, regular or no salt	13	3.91	135

Quaker Oats
rice cakes, lightly salted			
plain	1	0.3	35
multigrain	1	0.4	34
sesame	1	0.3	35
rice cakes, unsalted, plain	1	0.3	35

	Portion	Fiber (g)	Calories

□ **CREAM & CREAM SUBSTITUTES**
See MILK, MILK SUBSTITUTES,
& MILK PRODUCTS

□ **CROUTONS** *See* BREADCRUMBS,
CROUTONS, STUFFINGS,
& SEASONED COATINGS

□ **CUSTARDS** *See* DESSERTS: CUSTARDS,
GELATINS, & PUDDINGS

□ **DELI MEATS** *See* PROCESSED MEAT
& POULTRY PRODUCTS

□ **DESSERTS: CAKES, PASTRIES,
& PIES**

Cake

	Portion	Fiber (g)	Calories
banana, from mix, w/butter-cream icing	1.8 oz	tr •	181
Boston cream pie	3.9 oz	0.0 •	332
caramel, from mix	1.6 oz	0.1 •	173
w/caramel icing	1.9 oz	0.0 •	208
cheesecake, from mix	⅛ cake	0.1 •	300
chocolate, w/icing, from mix	1.3 oz cup-cake	0.1 •	129
fruitcake, light	1.4 oz	0.3 •	156
marble, from mix, w/white icing	1.8 oz	tr •	165
marble streusel, w/icing, from mix	2.3 oz	0.2 •	224
orange, homemade, w/icing	1.8 oz	tr •	183

Fiber figures marked with • refer to *crude* fiber. Unmarked fiber figures refer to *dietary* fiber.

	Portion	Fiber (g)	Calories
spice, from mix, w/vanilla icing	1.8 oz	tr •	176
white, from mix	2½ oz	0.1 •	219

Cake Icing

caramel	1.4 oz	0.0 •	140
chocolate	1.4 oz	tr •	148
coconut	1.4 oz	0.4 •	140
white, fluffy	0.6 oz	0.0 •	70

Fruit Bettys, Cobblers, & Crisps

apple brown Betty	½ c	0.7 •	211
apple crisp	½ c	0.4 •	302
peach cobbler	⅓ c	0.2 •	160
peach crisp	½ c	0.3 •	249

Pie

pie crusts *See* BAKING INGREDI- ENTS			
pineapple cheese, homemade	5.6 oz	0.1 •	270
shoofly, homemade	3.9 oz	0.1 •	441

❑ DESSERTS: CUSTARDS, GELATINS, & PUDDINGS

Custard

plain			
boiled, homemade	½ c	0.0 •	164
from mix	½ c	0.0 •	161

Gelatin

Bavarian (w/whipped cream)			
chocolate	1 serving	0.4 •	347
strawberry	1 serving	0.5 •	277

Pudding

butterscotch, homemade	½ c	0.0 •	207
lemon snow, homemade	½ c	0.0 •	114

	Portion	Fiber (g)	Calories
Rennin Dessert			
plain, homemade	½ c	0.0 •	113
chocolate, from mix			
prepared w/whole milk	½ c	0.1 •	127
prepared w/skim milk	½ c	0.1 •	95
fruit vanilla, from mix			
prepared w/whole milk	½ c	0.1 •	140
prepared w/skim milk	½ c	0.1 •	88

❑ DESSERTS, FROZEN

Ice cream & ice milk contain no dietary fiber.

Frozen Pudding on a Stick

banana	1	tr •	94
butterscotch	1	tr •	94
chocolate	1	0.1 •	99
chocolate fudge	1	0.1 •	99
vanilla	1	tr •	93

Ice Cream Cones

ice cream cone (cone only)	1	tr •	45

❑ EGGS & EGG SUBSTITUTES

Eggs from chickens & other fowl contain no dietary fiber.

Egg Substitute

frozen, containing egg white, corn oil, & nonfat dry milk	¼ c	0 •	96
liquid, containing egg white, soybean oil, & soy protein	1 c	0 •	211

Fiber figures marked with • refer to *crude* fiber. Unmarked fiber figures refer to *dietary* fiber.

	Portion	Fiber (g)	Calories
powder, containing egg white solids, whole egg solids, sweet whey solids, nonfat dry milk, & soy protein	0.7 oz	0 •	88

❑ ENTREES & MAIN COURSES, CANNED

chili & bean products *See* LEGUMES & LEGUME PRODUCTS; SOYBEANS & SOYBEAN PRODUCTS

▪ BRAND NAME

Van Camp's

Noodle Weenee	1 c	0.5 •	245
tamales w/sauce	1 c	2.2 •	293

❑ FAST FOODS

▪ BRAND NAME

Church's Fried Chicken
SIDE DISHES

corn, w/butter oil	1 ear	0.6 •	237
french fries, w/salt	1 regular serving	0.6 •	138

Pizza Hut
HAND-TOSSED PIZZA

cheese	2 slices	7	518
pepperoni	2 slices	6	500
Supreme	2 slices	7	540
Super Supreme	2 slices	7	556

PAN PIZZA

cheese	2 slices	5	492
pepperoni	2 slices	5	540

	Portion	Fiber (g)	Calories
Supreme	2 slices	7	589
Super Supreme	2 slices	6	563
PERSONAL PAN PIZZA			
pepperoni	2 slices	8	675
Supreme	2 slices	9	647
THIN 'N CRISPY PIZZA			
cheese	2 slices	4	398
pepperoni	2 slices	4	413
Supreme	2 slices	5	459
Super Supreme	2 slices	5	463

❏ FATS, OILS, & SHORTENINGS
See also BUTTER

Animal & vegetable fats, oils, & shortenings contain no dietary fiber.

❏ FISH *See* SEAFOOD & SEAFOOD PRODUCTS

❏ FLOURS & CORNMEALS
See also NUTS & NUT-BASED BUTTERS, FLOURS, MEALS, MILKS, PASTES, & POWDERS; SEEDS & SEED-BASED BUTTERS, FLOURS, & MEALS

barley flour	1 T	0.1 •	28
	1 c	0.8 •	401
buckwheat flour, dark	1 oz	0.4 •	92
carob flour	1 c	10.9 •	185
corn flour, sifted			
masa harina	⅓ c	0.7 •	137
masa trigo	⅓ c	0.1 •	149
white, tortilla, lime-treated	1 oz	0.9 •	103
yellow, tortilla, untreated	1 oz	0.4 •	101

Fiber figures marked with • refer to *crude* fiber. Unmarked fiber figures refer to *dietary* fiber.

	Portion	Fiber (g)	Calories
corn germ, toasted	1 oz	1.2 •	130
cornmeal, white, self-rising, dry	1 oz or ⅙ c	0.2 •	98
manioc (casava) flour	3½ oz	1.8 •	320
rice bran	1 oz	2.2 •	80
rice polish	1 oz	0.8 •	101
soy flour *See* SOYBEANS & SOYBEAN PRODUCTS			
wheat flour, enriched, bread, sifted	1 c	0.3 •	409
whole-wheat & soy flour	3½ oz	1.3 •	365
whole-wheat flour, from hard wheats	1 c	2.8 •	400
whole-wheat flour, straight, soft	3½ oz	0.4 •	364

▪ BRAND NAME

Argo
Argo & Kingsford's cornstarch	1 T	tr •	30

Arrowhead Mills
cornmeal, blue	2 oz	5.56	210
Ezekiel flour	2 oz	6.9	200
oat flour	2 oz	8.34	200
whole-wheat flour	2 oz	6.75	200

Aunt Jemima
CORNMEAL
bolted white, mix	⅙ c	0.2 •	99
bolted yellow, mix	⅙ c	0.1 •	97
buttermilk self-rising white, mix	3 T	0.3 •	101
enriched white	3 T	0.1 •	101
enriched yellow	3 T	0.1 •	101
self-rising white	⅙ c	0.2 •	98
self-rising white enriched bolted	⅙ c	0.3 •	99

FLOUR
enriched self-rising	¼ c	1.2 •	109

Quaker Oats
masa harina de maiz	⅓ c	0.6 •	137
masa trigo	⅓ c	0.9 •	149

❑ **FRANKFURTERS** *See* **PROCESSED MEAT & POULTRY PRODUCTS**

	Portion	Fiber (g)	Calories

❏ FRUIT, FRESH & PROCESSED

acerolas, raw	1 c	0.39 •	31
apples			
raw			
w/skin	1 fruit = 4.9 oz	1.06 •	81
w/out skin	1 fruit = 4½ oz	0.69 •	72
baked in microwave, w/out skin	½ c sliced	0.46 •	48
boiled, w/out skin	½ c sliced	0.46 •	46
canned, sweetened, unheated	½ c sliced	0.55 •	68
dehydrated, sulfured			
cooked	½ c	0.84 •	71
uncooked	½ c	1.23 •	104
dried, sulfured			
cooked, w/added sugar	½ c	0.88 •	116
cooked, w/out added sugar	½ c	0.86 •	72
uncooked	2¼ oz	1.84 •	155
	1 c	2.47 •	209
frozen, unsweetened			
heated	½ c sliced	0.56 •	48
unheated	½ c sliced	0.46 •	41
applesauce, canned			
sweetened	½ c	0.59 •	97
unsweetened	½ c	0.65 •	53
apricots			
raw	3 fruit = 3.7 oz	0.64 •	51
canned, w/skin			
in water	3 halves + 1¾ T liquid	0.36 •	22
in juice	3 halves + 1¾ T liquid	0.32 •	40
in extra-light syrup	3 halves + 1¾ T liquid	0.35 •	41

Fiber figures marked with • refer to *crude* fiber. Unmarked fiber figures refer to *dietary* fiber.

	Portion	Fiber (g)	Calories
apricots: canned, w/skin *(cont.)*			
in light syrup	3 halves + 1¾ T liquid	0.35 •	54
in heavy syrup	3 halves + 1¾ T liquid	0.34 •	70
canned, w/out skin			
in water	2 fruit + 2 T liquid	0.33 •	20
in heavy syrup	2 fruit + 2 T liquid	0.32 •	75
in extra-heavy syrup	2 fruit + 2 T liquid	0.31 •	87
dehydrated (low-moisture), sulfured			
cooked	½ c	1.93 •	156
uncooked	½ c	2.37 •	192
dried, sulfured			
cooked, w/added sugar	½ c halves	1.28 •	153
cooked, w/out added sugar	½ c halves	1.31 •	106
uncooked	10 halves	1.03 •	83
frozen, sweetened	½ c	0.73 •	119
avocados, raw			
all commercial varieties	1 fruit = 7.1 oz	4.24 •	324
	1 c puree	4.85 •	370
California	1 fruit = 6.1 oz	3.65 •	306
	1 c puree	4.85 •	407
Florida	1 fruit = 10.7 oz	6.41 •	339
	1 c puree	4.85 •	257
bananas			
raw	1 fruit = 4 oz	0.57 •	105
dehydrated (banana powder)	1 T	0.12 •	21
blackberries			
raw	½ c	2.95 •	37
canned, in heavy syrup	½ c	3.33 •	118
frozen, unsweetened	1 c	4.08 •	97
blueberries			
raw	1 c	1.88 •	82
canned, in heavy syrup	½ c	1.15 •	112
frozen			
sweetened	1 c	2.07 •	187
unsweetened	1 c	2.32 •	78

	Portion	Fiber (g)	Calories
boysenberries			
canned, in heavy syrup	½ c	2.43 •	113
frozen, unsweetened	1 c	3.56 •	66
breadfruit, raw	¼ small fruit = 3.4 oz	1.42 •	99
candied fruit *See* BAKING INGREDIENTS			
cantaloupe *See* melons, *below*			
carambolas, raw	1 fruit = 4½ oz	1.17 •	42
carissa plums, raw	1 fruit = 0.7 oz	0.18 •	12
casaba *See* melons, *below*			
cherimoyas, raw	1 fruit = 19¼ oz	12.03 •	515
cherries, sour, red			
raw	1 c w/pits	0.21 •	51
canned			
in water	½ c	0.12 •	43
in light syrup	½ c	0.13 •	94
in heavy syrup	½ c	0.13 •	116
in extra-heavy syrup	½ c	0.13 •	148
frozen, unsweetened	1 c	0.46 •	72
cherries, sweet			
raw	10 fruit = 2.4 oz	0.27 •	49
canned			
in water	½ c	0.25 •	57
in juice	½ c	0.28 •	68
in light syrup	½ c	0.40 •	85
in extra-heavy syrup	½ c	0.40 •	133
in heavy syrup	½ c	0.40 •	107
frozen, sweetened	1 c	1.04 •	232
Chinese gooseberries *See* kiwi fruit, *below*			
coconut *See* NUTS & NUT-BASED BUTTERS, FLOURS, MEALS, MILKS, PASTES, & POWDERS			
crabapples, raw	1 c sliced	0.66 •	83
cranberries, raw	1 c whole	1.14 •	46
cranberry sauce, canned, sweetened	½ c	0.41 •	209

Fiber figures marked with • refer to *crude* fiber. Unmarked fiber figures refer to *dietary* fiber.

	Portion	Fiber (g)	Calories
currants			
European, black, raw	½ c	1.34 •	36
red & white, raw	½ c	1.90 •	31
zante, dried	½ c	1.13 •	204
custard apples, raw	edible portion = 3½ oz	3.40 •	101
dates, domestic, dry	10 fruit = 2.9 oz	1.83 •	228
elderberries, raw	1 c	10.15 •	105
figs			
raw	1 medium fruit = 1¾ oz	0.60 •	37
canned			
in water	3 fruit + 1¾ T liquid	0.46 •	42
in light syrup	3 fruit + 1¾ T liquid	0.48 •	58
in heavy syrup	3 fruit + 1¾ T liquid	0.47 •	75
in extra-heavy syrup	3 fruit + 1¾ T liquid	0.46 •	91
dried			
cooked	½ c	2.63 •	140
uncooked	10 fruit = 6.6 oz	8.97 •	477
fruit cocktail, canned			
in water	½ c	0.57 •	40
in juice	½ c	0.43 •	56
in extra-light syrup	½ c	0.57 •	55
in light syrup	½ c	0.57 •	72
in heavy syrup	½ c	0.57 •	93
in extra-heavy syrup	½ c	0.57 •	115
fruit salad, canned			
in water	½ c	0.76 •	37
in juice	½ c	0.44 •	62
in light syrup	½ c	0.77 •	73
in heavy syrup	½ c	0.77 •	94
in extra-heavy syrup	½ c	0.77 •	114
fruit salad, tropical, canned, in heavy syrup	½ c	0.57 •	110
gooseberries			
raw	1 c	2.85 •	67
canned, in light syrup	½ c	1.51 •	93
grandillas See passion fruit, below			

	Portion	Fiber (g)	Calories
grapefruit			
raw, pink & red	½ fruit = 4.3 oz	0.25 •	37
raw, white	½ fruit = 4.2 oz	0.24 •	39
canned			
in water	½ c	0.40 •	44
in juice	½ c	0.22 •	46
in light syrup	½ c	0.41 •	76
grapes			
American type, raw	10 fruit = 0.8 oz	0.18 •	15
European type, raw	10 fruit = 1.8 oz	0.23 •	36
Thompson seedless, canned			•
in water	½ c	0.25 •	48
in heavy syrup, solids & liquids	½ c	0.25 •	94
groundcherries, raw	½ c	1.96 •	37
guava sauce, cooked	½ c	2.37 •	43
guavas			
common, raw	1 fruit = 3.2 oz	5.04 •	45
strawberry, raw	1 fruit = 0.2 oz	0.38 •	4
honeydew See melons, below			
jackfruit, raw	edible portion = 3½ oz	1.00 •	94
jujubes			
raw	edible portion = 3½ oz	1.40 •	79
dried	edible portion = 3½ oz	3.00 •	287
kiwi fruit, raw	1 medium fruit = 2.7 oz	0.84 •	46
kumquats, raw	1 fruit = 0.7 oz	0.70 •	12
lemons, raw, w/out peel	1 medium fruit = 2 oz	0.23 •	17

Fiber figures marked with • refer to *crude* fiber. Unmarked fiber figures refer to *dietary* fiber.

	Portion	Fiber (g)	Calories
limes, raw	1 fruit = 2.4 oz	0.34 •	20
litchis *See* lychees, *below*			
longans			
raw	1 fruit = 0.1 oz	0.01 •	2
dried	edible portion = 3½ oz	2.00 •	286
loquats, raw	1 fruit = 0.3 oz	0.05 •	5
lychees			
raw	1 fruit = 0.3 oz	0.02 •	6
dried	edible portion = 3½ oz	1.40 •	277
mammy apples, raw	1 fruit = 29.8 oz	8.46 •	431
mangos, raw	1 fruit = 7.3 oz	1.73 •	135
melons			
cantaloupe, raw	½ fruit = 9.4 oz	0.97 •	94
	1 c cubed	0.58 •	57
casaba, raw	1/10 fruit = 5.8 oz	0.82 •	43
	1 c cubed	0.85 •	45
honeydew, raw	1/10 fruit = 4½ oz	0.77 •	46
	1 c cubed	1.02 •	60
muskmelons *See* melons: cantaloupe, *above*			
mixed fruit			
canned, in heavy syrup, solids & liquids	½ c	0.51 •	92
dried	11 oz	8.48 •	712
mulberries, raw	10 fruit = ½ oz	0.14 •	7
muskmelons *See* melons: cantaloupe, *above*			
natal plums *See* carissa plums, *above*			
nectarines, raw	1 fruit = 4.8 oz	0.54 •	67
oheloberries, raw	10 fruit = 0.4 oz	0.15 •	3
oranges, raw, w/out peel			
California, navels	1 fruit = 4.9 oz	0.64 •	65

	Portion	Fiber (g)	Calories
California, Valencias	1 fruit = 4.3 oz	0.61 •	59
Florida	1 fruit = 5.3 oz	0.52 •	69
other commercial varieties	1 fruit = 4.6 oz	0.56 •	62
papayas, raw	1 fruit = 10.7 oz	2.35 •	117
passion fruit, purple, raw	1 fruit = 0.6 oz	1.97 •	18
peaches			
raw	1 fruit = 3.1 oz	0.56 •	37
canned, clingstone			
in water	1 half + 1⅔ T liquid	0.24 •	18
in extra-light syrup	1 half + 1⅔ T liquid	0.15 •	32
in light syrup	1 half + 1¾ T liquid	0.24 •	44
canned, clingstone & freestone			
in juice	1 half + 1⅔ T liquid	0.19 •	34
in heavy syrup	1 half + 1¾ T liquid	0.24 •	60
canned, freestone, in extra-heavy syrup	1 half + 1¾ T liquid	0.23 •	77
dehydrated (low-moisture), sulfured			
cooked	½ c	1.97 •	161
uncooked	½ c	2.30 •	188
dried, sulfured			
cooked, w/added sugar	½ c halves	1.16 •	139
cooked, w/out added sugar	½ c halves	1.21 •	99
uncooked	10 halves	3.81 •	311
frozen, sweetened	1 c sliced, thawed	1.00 •	235
peaches, spiced, canned, in heavy syrup	1 fruit + 2 T liquid	0.22 •	66

Fiber figures marked with • refer to *crude* fiber. Unmarked fiber figures refer to *dietary* fiber.

	Portion	Fiber (g)	Calories
pears			
raw	1 fruit = 5.8 oz	2.32 •	98
canned			
in water	1 half + 1⅔ T liquid	0.47 •	22
in juice	1 half + 1⅔ T liquid	0.38 •	38
in extra-light syrup	1 half + 1⅔ T liquid	0.46 •	36
in light syrup	1 half + 1¾ T liquid	215	45
in heavy syrup	1 half + 1¾ T liquid	0.46 •	58
in extra-heavy syrup	1 half + 1¾ T liquid	0.45 •	77
dried, sulfured			
cooked, w/out added sugar	½ c halves	3.53 •	163
cooked, w/added sugar	½ c halves	3.67 •	196
uncooked	10 halves	9.95 •	459
persimmons			
Japanese			
raw	1 fruit = 5.9 oz	2.49 •	118
dried	1 fruit = 1.2 oz	1.23 •	93
native, raw	1 fruit = 0.9 oz	0.38 •	32
pineapple			
raw	1 c diced	0.84 •	77
canned			
in water	1 slice + 1¼ T liquid	0.26 •	19
	1 c tidbits	1.11 •	79
in juice	1 slice + 1¼ T liquid	0.20 •	35
	1 c chunks or tidbits	0.87 •	150
in light syrup	1 slice + 1¼ T liquid	0.26 •	30
	1 c	1.12 •	131

	Portion	Fiber (g)	Calories
in heavy syrup	1 slice + 1¼ T liquid	0.25 •	45
	1 c chunks, tidbits, or crushed	1.11 •	199
in extra-heavy syrup	1 slice + 1¼ T liquid	0.25 •	48
	1 c chunks or crushed	1.12 •	217
frozen, sweetened	1 slice = 3 oz	0.45 •	42
	½ c chunks	0.37 •	104
pitangas, raw	1 fruit = 0.2 oz	0.04 •	2
	1 c	1.04 •	57
plantains, raw	1 fruit = 6.3 oz	0.90 •	218
plums, purple			
raw	1 fruit = 2.3 oz	0.40 •	36
canned			
in water	3 fruit + 2 T liquid	0.24 •	39
	1 c	0.62 •	102
in juice	3 fruit + 2 T liquid	0.25 •	55
	1 c	0.66 •	146
in light syrup	3 fruit + 2¾ T liquid	0.45 •	83
	1 c	0.85 •	158
in heavy syrup	3 fruit + 2¾ T liquid	0.44 •	119
	1 c	0.85 •	230
in extra-heavy syrup	3 fruit + 2¾ T liquid	0.43 •	135
	1 c	0.84 •	265
pomegranates, raw	1 fruit = 5.4 oz	0.31 •	104
prickly pears, raw	1 fruit = 3.6 oz	1.87 •	42

Fiber figures marked with • refer to *crude* fiber. Unmarked fiber figures refer to *dietary* fiber.

	Portion	Fiber (g)	Calories
prunes			
canned, in heavy syrup	5 fruit + 2 T liquid	0.60 •	90
	1 c	1.63 •	245
dehydrated (low-moisture)			
cooked	½ c	1.35 •	158
uncooked	½ c	1.91 •	224
dried			
cooked, w/added sugar	½ c	1.02 •	147
cooked, w/out added sugar	½ c	0.97 •	113
uncooked	10 fruit = 3 oz	1.72 •	201
	1 c	3.29 •	385
pummelos, raw	1 fruit = 21.4 oz	1.10 •	228
	1 c sections	0.34 •	71
quinces, raw	1 fruit = 3.2 oz	1.56 •	53
raisins			
golden seedless	1 c not packed	2.08 •	437
	1 c packed	2.36 •	498
seeded	1 c not packed	0.97 •	428
	1 c packed	1.11 •	488
seedless	1 c not packed	1.85 •	434
	1 c packed	2.11 •	494
raspberries, red			
raw	1 c	3.69 •	61
frozen, sweetened	1 c	5.53 •	256
	10 oz pkg	6.28 •	291
rhubarb			
raw	½ c diced	0.43 •	13
frozen, cooked, w/added sugar	½ c	0.96 •	139
rose apples, raw	edible portion = 3½ oz	1.10 •	25
roselles, raw	1 c	0.65 •	28
sapodillas, raw	1 fruit = 6 oz	2.38 •	140
sapotes, raw	1 fruit = 7.9 oz	4.28 •	301
soursops, raw	1 fruit = 22 oz	6.88 •	416

starfruit *See* carambolas, *above*

	Portion	Fiber (g)	Calories
strawberries			
raw	1 c	0.79 •	45
frozen, sweetened			
whole	1 c	1.50 •	200
	10 oz pkg	1.68 •	223
sliced	1 c	1.57 •	245
	10 oz pkg	1.75 •	273
frozen, unsweetened	1 c	1.18 •	52
sugar apples, raw	1 fruit = 5½ oz	2.28 •	146
Surinam cherries *See* pitangas, *above*			
sweetsops *See* sugar apples, *above*			
tamarinds, raw	1 fruit = 0.1 oz	0.10 •	5
tangerines			
raw	1 fruit = 3 oz	0.28 •	37
canned			
in juice, solids & liquids	½ c	0.13 •	46
in light syrup, solids & liquids	½ c	0.16 •	76
watermelon, raw	1/16 fruit = 17 oz	1.45 •	152
	1 c diced	0.48 •	50
West Indian cherries *See* acerolas, *above*			

■ **BRAND NAME**

Birds Eye

mixed fruit in syrup	5 oz	0.8	120
red raspberries in lite syrup	5 oz	4.3	100
strawberries, halved, in lite syrup	5 oz	2.1	90
strawberries, halved, in syrup	5 oz	2.1	120

❑ FRUIT SPREADS

Fruit Butters

Fiber figures marked with • refer to *crude* fiber. Unmarked fiber figures refer to *dietary* fiber.

	Portion	Fiber (g)	Calories
apple	1 T	0.2 •	37
guava	1 T	0.0 •	39

Jams

| average, all varieties, regular | 1 T | 0.1 • | 55 |

Jellies

| average, all varieties, regular | 1 T | 0.0 • | 55 |

Marmalades

| citrus | 1 T | 0.0 • | 51 |

□ **GELATIN & GELATIN DESSERTS**
See DESSERTS: CUSTARDS, GELATINS,
& PUDDINGS

□ **GRAINS** *See* RICE & GRAINS,
PLAIN & PREPARED

□ **GRAVIES** *See* SAUCES & GRAVIES

□ **HAM** *See* PORK, FRESH & CURED

□ **HERBS & SPICES** *See* SEASONINGS

□ **HONEY** *See* SUGARS & SWEETENERS

□ **HOT DOGS** *See* PROCESSED MEAT
& POULTRY PRODUCTS

□ **ICE CREAM & ICE MILK**
See DESSERTS, FROZEN

	Portion	Fiber (g)	Calories

❑ **INFANT & TODDLER FOODS**

Baked Products

pretzels	1	0.0 •	24
	1 oz	0.1 •	113
teething biscuits	1	0.1 •	43
	1 oz	0.1 •	111
zwieback	1	0.0 •	30
	1 oz	0.1 •	121

Cereals, Hot & Cold

barley			
dry	½ oz	0.2 •	52
	1 T	0.0 •	9
w/whole milk	1 oz	0.1 •	31
cereal & egg yolks			
strained	about 4½ oz	0.2 •	66
	1 oz	0.0 •	15
junior	about 7½ oz	0.2 •	110
	1 oz	0.0 •	15
cereal, egg yolks, & bacon			
high protein			
dry	½ oz	0.3 •	51
	1 T	0.1 •	9
w/whole milk	1 oz	0.1 •	31
high protein w/apple & orange			
dry	½ oz	0.2 •	53
	1 T	0.0 •	9
w/whole milk	1 oz	0.1 •	32
mixed			
dry	½ oz	0.1 •	54
	1 T	0.0 •	9
w/whole milk	1 oz	0.0 •	32
mixed w/applesauce & bananas			
strained	about 4.8 oz	0.4 •	111
	1 oz	0.1 •	23
junior	about 7.8 oz	0.1 •	183
	1 oz	0.1 •	24

Fiber figures marked with • refer to *crude* fiber. Unmarked fiber figures refer to *dietary* fiber.

	Portion	Fiber (g)	Calories
mixed w/bananas			
dry	½ oz	0.1 •	56
	1 T	0.0 •	9
w/whole milk	1 oz	0.0 •	33
oatmeal			
dry	½ oz	0.2 •	56
	1 T	0.0 •	10
w/whole milk	1 oz	0.1 •	33
oatmeal w/applesauce & bananas			
strained	about 4.8 oz	1.0 •	99
	1 oz	0.2 •	21
junior	about 7.8 oz	0.9 •	165
	1 oz	0.1 •	21
oatmeal w/bananas			
dry	½ oz	0.1 •	56
	1 T	0.0 •	9
w/whole milk	1 oz	0.0 •	33
rice			
dry	½ oz	0.1 •	56
	1 T	0.0 •	9
w/whole milk	1 oz	0.0 •	33
rice w/applesauce & bananas,	about 4.8 oz	0.2 •	107
strained	1 oz	0.0 •	23
rice w/bananas			
dry	½ oz	0.1 •	57
	1 T	0.0 •	10
w/whole milk	1 oz	0.0 •	33
rice w/mixed fruit, junior	about 7.8 oz	0.5 •	186
	1 oz	0.1 •	24

Desserts

	Portion	Fiber (g)	Calories
cherry vanilla pudding			
strained	about 4.8 oz	0.2 •	91
	1 oz	0.0 •	19
junior	about 7.8 oz	0.3 •	152
	1 oz	0.0 •	20
cottage cheese w/pineapple			
strained	about 4.8 oz	1.7 •	94
	1 oz	0.4 •	20
junior	about 7.8 oz	2.1 •	172
	1 oz	0.3 •	22

	Portion	Fiber (g)	Calories
Dutch apple			
strained	about 4.8 oz	0.3 •	92
	1 oz	0.1 •	19
junior	about 7.8 oz	0.6 •	151
	1 oz	0.1 •	19
fruit dessert			
strained	about 4.8 oz	0.3 •	79
	1 oz	0.1 •	17
junior	about 7.8 oz	0.7 •	138
	1 oz	0.1 •	18
orange pudding, strained	about 4.8 oz	0.5 •	108
	1 oz	0.1 •	23
pineapple pudding			
strained	about 4½ oz	0.9 •	104
	1 oz	0.2 •	23
junior	about 7.8 oz	1.7 •	192
	1 oz	0.2 •	25

Dinners, High in Meat or Cheese

	Portion	Fiber (g)	Calories
beef w/vegetables			
strained	about 4½ oz	0.4 •	96
	1 oz	0.1 •	21
junior	about 4½ oz	0.3 •	108
	1 oz	0.1 •	24
chicken w/vegetables			
strained	about 4½ oz	0.3 •	100
	1 oz	0.1 •	22
junior	about 4½ oz	0.3 •	117
	1 oz	0.1 •	26
cottage cheese w/pineapple, strained	about 4.8 oz	1.2 •	157
	1 oz	0.3 •	33
ham w/vegetables			
strained	about 4½ oz	0.3 •	97
	1 oz	0.1 •	21
junior	about 4½ oz	0.2 •	98
	1 oz	0.1 •	22
turkey w/vegetables			
strained	about 4½ oz	0.1 •	111
	1 oz	0.0 •	25

Fiber figures marked with • refer to *crude* fiber. Unmarked fiber figures refer to *dietary* fiber.

	Portion	Fiber (g)	Calories
turkey w/vegetables *(cont.)*			
junior	about 4½ oz	0.3 •	115
	1 oz	0.1 •	25
veal w/vegetables			
strained	about 4½ oz	0.4 •	89
	1 oz	0.1 •	20
junior	about 4½ oz	0.2 •	93
	1 oz	0.1 •	21

Dinners, Regular

	Portion	Fiber (g)	Calories
beef & egg noodles			
strained	about 4½ oz	0.4 •	68
	1 oz	0.1 •	15
junior	about 7½ oz	0.4 •	122
	1 oz	0.1 •	16
beef & rice, toddler	about 6.2 oz	0.5 •	146
	1 oz	0.1 •	23
beef lasagna, toddler	about 6.2 oz	0.4 •	137
	1 oz	0.1 •	22
beef stew, toddler	about 6.2 oz	0.5 •	90
	1 oz	0.1 •	14
chicken & noodles			
strained	about 4½ oz	0.4 •	67
	1 oz	0.1 •	15
junior	about 7½ oz	1.3 •	109
	1 oz	0.2 •	15
chicken soup, cream of, strained	about 4½ oz	0.4 •	74
	1 oz	0.1 •	16
chicken stew, toddler	about 6 oz	0.5 •	132
	1 oz	0.1 •	22
macaroni & cheese			
junior	about 7½ oz	0.2 •	130
	1 oz	0.0 •	17
strained	about 4½ oz	0.1 •	76
	1 oz	0.0 •	17
macaroni, tomato, & beef			
strained	about 4½ oz	0.5 •	71
	1 oz	0.1 •	16
junior	about 7½ oz	0.6 •	125
	1 oz	0.1 •	17
spaghetti, tomato, & meat			
junior	about 7½ oz	0.9 •	135
	1 oz	0.1 •	18

	Portion	Fiber (g)	Calories
toddler	about 6.2 oz	0.7 •	133
	1 oz	0.1 •	21
split peas & ham, junior	about 7½ oz	0.6 •	152
	1 oz	0.1 •	20
turkey & rice			
strained	about 4½ oz	0.1 •	63
	1 oz	0.0 •	14
junior	about 7½ oz	0.4 •	104
	1 oz	0.1 •	14
vegetables & bacon			
strained	about 4½ oz	0.5 •	88
	1 oz	0.1 •	19
junior	about 7½ oz	0.4 •	150
	1 oz	0.1 •	20
vegetables & beef			
strained	about 4½ oz	0.3 •	67
	1 oz	0.1 •	15
junior	about 7½ oz	0.4 •	113
	1 oz	0.1 •	15
vegetables & chicken			
strained	about 4½ oz	0.3 •	55
	1 oz	0.1 •	12
junior	about 7½ oz	0.4 •	106
	1 oz	0.1 •	14
vegetables & ham			
junior	about 7½ oz	0.4 •	110
	1 oz	0.1 •	15
strained	about 4½ oz	0.2 •	62
	1 oz	0.1 •	14
vegetables & lamb			
strained	about 4½ oz	0.4 •	67
	1 oz	0.1 •	15
junior	about 7½ oz	0.4 •	108
	1 oz	0.1 •	14
vegetables & liver			
strained	about 4½ oz	0.2 •	50
	1 oz	0.1 •	11
junior	about 7½ oz	0.6 •	93
	1 oz	0.1 •	12

Fiber figures marked with • refer to *crude* fiber. Unmarked fiber figures refer to *dietary* fiber.

	Portion	Fiber (g)	Calories
vegetables & turkey			
strained	about 4½ oz	0.3 •	54
	1 oz	0.1 •	12
junior	about 7½ oz	0.4 •	101
	1 oz	0.1 •	13
toddler	about 6.2 oz	0.9 •	141
	1 oz	0.1 •	23
vegetables, noodles, & chicken			
strained	about 4½ oz	0.2 •	81
	1 oz	0.1 •	18
junior	about 7½ oz	0.4 •	137
	1 oz	0.1 •	18
vegetables, noodles, & turkey			
strained	about 4½ oz	0.3 •	56
	1 oz	0.1 •	12
junior	about 7½ oz	0.5 •	110
	1 oz	0.1 •	15

Fruit
See also Desserts, *above*

	Portion	Fiber (g)	Calories
apple blueberry			
strained	about 4.8 oz	0.3 •	82
	1 oz	0.1 •	17
junior	about 7.8 oz	0.4 •	137
	1 oz	0.1 •	18
applesauce			
strained	about 4½ oz	0.7 •	53
	1 oz	0.2 •	12
junior	about 7½ oz	1.2 •	79
	1 oz	0.2 •	11
applesauce & apricots			
strained	about 4.8 oz	0.9 •	60
	1 oz	0.2 •	13
junior	about 7.8 oz	1.5 •	104
	1 oz	0.2 •	13
apricots w/tapioca			
strained	about 4.8 oz	0.4 •	80
	1 oz	0.1 •	17
junior	about 7.8 oz	1.0 •	139
	1 oz	0.1 •	18
bananas w/tapioca			
strained	about 4.8 oz	0.2 •	77
	1 oz	0.0 •	16
junior	about 7.8 oz	0.4 •	147
	1 oz	0.1 •	19

	Portion	Fiber (g)	Calories
guava & papaya w/tapioca, strained	about ½ oz	1.3 •	80
	1 oz	0.3 •	18
guava w/tapioca, strained	about 4½ oz	0.7 •	86
	1 oz	0.2 •	19
mango w/tapioca, strained	about 4.8 oz	0.2 •	109
	1 oz	0.0 •	23
papaya & applesauce w/tapioca, strained	about 4½ oz	0.5 •	89
	1 oz	0.1 •	20
peaches			
strained	about 4.8 oz	1.0 •	96
	1 oz	0.2 •	20
junior	about 7.8 oz	1.6 •	157
	1 oz	0.2 •	20
pears & pineapple			
strained	about 4½ oz	0.3 •	52
	1 oz	0.1 •	12
junior	about 7½ oz	0.5 •	93
	1 oz	0.1 •	12
prunes w/tapioca			
strained	about 4.8 oz	0.4 •	94
	1 oz	0.1 •	20
junior	about 7.8 oz	0.7 •	155
	1 oz	0.1 •	20

Meats & Egg Yolks

	Portion	Fiber (g)	Calories
beef w/beef heart, strained	about 3½ oz	0.1 •	93
	1 oz	0.0 •	27
chicken sticks, junior	1 stick = 0.35 oz	0.0 •	19
	2½ oz	0.1 •	134
meat sticks, junior	1 stick = 0.35 oz	0.0 •	18
	2½ oz	0.1 •	130
turkey sticks, junior	1 stick = 0.35 oz	0.0 •	18
	2½ oz	0.4 •	129
veal			
strained	about 3½ oz	0.1 •	100
	1 oz	0.0 •	29

Fiber figures marked with • refer to *crude* fiber. Unmarked fiber figures refer to *dietary* fiber.

	Portion	Fiber (g)	Calories
veal *(cont.)*			
junior	about 3½ oz	0.2 •	109
	1 oz	0.0 •	31
Vegetables			
beans, green, plain			
strained	about 4½ oz	1.3 •	32
	1 oz	0.3 •	7
junior	about 7.3 oz	2.0 •	51
	1 oz	0.3 •	7
beets, strained	about 4½ oz	1.0 •	43
	1 oz	0.2 •	10
carrots, plain			
strained	about 4½ oz	1.0 •	34
	1 oz	0.2 •	8
junior	about 7½ oz	1.7 •	67
	1 oz	0.2 •	9
corn, creamed			
strained	about 4½ oz	0.4 •	73
	1 oz	0.1 •	16
junior	about 7½ oz	0.2 •	138
	1 oz	0.0 •	18
garden vegetables, strained	about 4½ oz	1.2 •	48
	1 oz	0.3 •	11
mixed vegetables			
strained	about 4½ oz	0.5 •	52
	1 oz	0.1 •	11
junior	about 7½ oz	1.1 •	88
	1 oz	0.1 •	12
peas			
plain, strained	about 4½ oz	1.5 •	52
	1 oz	0.3 •	11
creamed, strained	about 4½ oz	0.5 •	68
	1 oz	0.1 •	15
spinach, creamed			
strained	about 4½ oz	0.6 •	48
	1 oz	0.1 •	11
junior	about 7½ oz	1.1 •	90
	1 oz	0.1 •	12
squash, plain			
strained	about 4½ oz	0.9 •	30
	1 oz	0.2 •	7
junior	about 7½ oz	1.5 •	51
	1 oz	0.2 •	7

	Portion	Fiber (g)	Calories
sweet potatoes, plain			
strained	about 4.8 oz	0.9 •	77
	1 oz	0.2 •	16
junior	about 7.8 oz	1.4 •	133
	1 oz	0.2 •	17

■ BRAND NAME

Gerber
BAKED GOODS

animal crackers	4	0.07	50
animal-shaped cookies	2	0.16	60
arrowroot cookies	2	0.06	50
pretzels	2	0.19	50
Toddler Biter biscuits	1	0.08	50
zwieback toast	2	0.13	60

CHUNKY PRODUCTS

Homestyle noodles & beef	6 oz	0.68	150
noodles & chicken w/carrots & peas	6 oz	1	110
rice w/beef & tomato sauce	6¼ oz	0.89	140
saucy rice w/chicken	6 oz	0.68	120
spaghetti tomato sauce & beef	6¼ oz	1.23	160
vegetables & beef	6¼ oz	0.89	130
vegetables & chicken	6¼ oz	1.06	140
vegetables & ham	6¼ oz	0.89	130
vegetables & turkey	6¼ oz	0.89	120

DRY CEREALS, READY-TO-SERVE

barley	½ oz dry	0.91	60
	½ oz dry + 2.4 fl oz milk	0.91	100
high protein	½ oz dry	0.57	50
	½ oz dry + 2.4 fl oz milk	0.57	100
w/apple & orange	½ oz dry	0.51	60
	½ oz dry + 2.4 fl oz milk	0.51	100

Fiber figures marked with • refer to *crude* fiber. Unmarked fiber figures refer to *dietary* fiber.

	Portion	Fiber (g)	Calories
mixed	½ oz dry	0.37	50
	½ oz dry + 2.4 fl oz milk	0.37	100
w/banana	½ oz dry	0.37	60
	½ oz dry + 2.4 fl oz milk	0.37	100
oatmeal	½ oz dry	0.62	60
	½ oz dry + 2.4 fl oz milk	0.62	100
w/banana	½ oz dry	0.48	60
	½ oz dry + 2.4 fl oz milk	0.48	100
rice	½ oz dry	0.11	60
	½ oz dry + 2.4 fl oz milk	0.11	100
w/banana	½ oz dry	0.18	60
	½ oz dry + 2.4 fl oz milk	0.18	100

FIRST FOODS

Fruit

applesauce	2½ oz	0.71	40
bananas	2½ oz	0.43	60
peaches	2½ oz	0.50	30
pears	2½ oz	1.42	40
prunes	2½ oz	0.5	70

Vegetables

carrots	2½ oz	0.71	40
green beans	2½ oz	0.92	20
peas	2½ oz	1.27	40
squash	2½ oz	1.13	20
sweet potatoes	2½ oz	0.50	50

JUNIOR FOODS

Cereals w/Fruit

mixed w/applesauce & bananas	6 oz	1.02	140
oatmeal w/applesauce & bananas	6 oz	1.19	130

	Portion	Fiber (g)	Calories
rice w/mixed fruit	6 oz	0.51	140
Desserts			
Dutch apple	6 oz	2.55	130
fruit	6 oz	0.34	130
Hawaiian Delight	6 oz	0.51	150
peach cobbler	6 oz	0.51	130
Dinners, Lean Meat			
beef w/vegetables	4½ oz	0.51	100
chicken w/vegetables	4½ oz	0.51	90
ham w/vegetables	4½ oz	0.51	110
turkey w/vegetables	4½ oz	0.38	100
Dinners, Regular			
beef egg noodle	6 oz	0.68	120
chicken noodle	6 oz	0.68	100
macaroni tomato beef	6 oz	0.85	110
spaghetti tomato sauce beef	6 oz	0.85	120
split peas ham	6 oz	1.36	130
turkey rice	6 oz	0.68	110
vegetable bacon	6 oz	1.19	140
vegetable beef	6 oz	0.85	110
vegetable chicken	6 oz	0.68	100
vegetable ham	6 oz	0.68	120
vegetable lamb	6 oz	0.68	120
vegetable turkey	6 oz	0.68	100
Fruit			
apple blueberry	6 oz	1.7	80
applesauce	6 oz	1.36	90
apricots w/tapioca	6 oz	0.51	130
bananas w/pineapple & tapioca	6 oz	0.68	90
bananas w/tapioca	6 oz	0.68	140
peaches	6 oz	1.02	110
pear pineapple	6 oz	3.06	100
pears	6 oz	3.23	100
plums w/tapioca	6 oz	0.68	130

Fiber figures marked with • refer to *crude* fiber. Unmarked fiber figures refer to *dietary* fiber.

	Portion	Fiber (g)	Calories
Meats			
beef	2½ oz	0.07	80
ham	2½ oz	0.07	90
Vegetables			
carrots	6 oz	1.36	50
creamed green beans	6 oz	1.19	80
mixed vegetables	6 oz	1.70	70
peas	6 oz	3.23	90
squash	6 oz	1.87	60
sweet potatoes	6 oz	1.36	110
STRAINED FOODS			
Cereals w/Fruit			
mixed w/applesauce & bananas	4½ oz	0.77	100
oatmeal w/applesauce & bananas	4½ oz	1.02	100
rice w/applesauce & bananas	4½ oz	0.38	100
Desserts			
banana apple	4½ oz	0.38	90
cherry vanilla pudding	4½ oz	0.13	90
chocolate custard pudding	4½ oz	0.13	110
Dutch apple	4½ oz	0.51	100
fruit	4½ oz	0.26	100
Hawaiian Delight	4½ oz	0.13	120
orange pudding	4½ oz	0.13	110
peach cobbler	4½ oz	0.38	100
vanilla custard pudding	4½ oz	0.13	100
Dinners, Lean Meat			
beef w/vegetables	4½ oz	0.26	90
chicken w/vegetables	4½ oz	0.26	90
ham w/vegetables	4½ oz	0.26	100
turkey w/vegetables	4½ oz	0.26	100
Dinners, Regular			
beef egg noodle	4½ oz	0.51	90
chicken noodle	4½ oz	0.38	90
macaroni cheese	4½ oz	0.38	90
macaroni tomato beef	4½ oz	0.51	80
turkey rice	4½ oz	0.38	80

	Portion	Fiber (g)	Calories
vegetable bacon	4½ oz	0.77	100
vegetable beef	4½ oz	0.51	90
vegetable chicken	4½ oz	0.51	80
vegetable ham	4½ oz	0.51	80
vegetable lamb	4½ oz	0.51	90
vegetable liver	4½ oz	0.51	60
vegetable turkey	4½ oz	0.38	70

Fruit & Tropical Fruit

apple blueberry	4½ oz	1.28	60
applesauce	4½ oz	1.02	60
applesauce apricot	4½ oz	1.28	70
apricots w/tapioca	4½ oz	0.38	90
bananas w/pineapple & tapioca	4½ oz	0.38	60
bananas w/tapioca	4½ oz	0.51	110
guava w/tapioca	4½ oz	0.90	90
mango w/tapioca	4½ oz	0.38	90
papaya w/tapioca	4½ oz	0.38	80
peaches	4½ oz	0.77	90
pear pineapple	4½ oz	1.92	80
pears	4½ oz	1.53	80
plums w/tapioca	4½ oz	0.51	90
prunes w/tapioca	4½ oz	0.90	100

Juices

apple	4.2 oz	0.13	60
apple apricot	4.2 oz	0.26	60
apple banana	4.2 oz	0.13	70
apple cherry	4.2 oz	0.13	60
apple grape	4.2 oz	0.13	60
apple peach	4.2 oz	0.13	60
apple pineapple	4.2 oz	0.13	60
apple prune	4.2 oz	0.13	70
mixed fruit	4.2 oz	0.13	70
orange	4.2 oz	0.13	70

Vegetables

beets	4½ oz	1.15	60
carrots	4½ oz	1.02	40
creamed corn	4½ oz	0.51	80
creamed spinach	4½ oz	1.02	60

Fiber figures marked with • refer to *crude* fiber. Unmarked fiber figures refer to *dietary* fiber.

	Portion	Fiber (g)	Calories
garden vegetables	4½ oz	1.92	50
green beans	4½ oz	1.40	50
mixed vegetables	4½ oz	0.77	60
peas	4½ oz	2.30	60
squash	4½ oz	1.28	40
sweet potatoes	4½ oz	0.90	80

TODDLER FOODS

Cereals

Toasted Oat Rings	½ oz dry	0.60	60
	½ oz dry + 2.7 fl oz milk	0.60	110

Juices

apple	4 oz	0.13	60
apple & berry	4 oz	0.13	60
apple cherry	4 oz	0.13	60
apple grape	4 oz	0.13	60
Fruits of the Sun	4 oz	0.13	60
Fruits-A-Plenty	4 oz	0.13	60
mixed fruit	4 oz	0.13	60
pear	4 oz	0.13	60

Meat & Poultry Sticks

chicken	2½ oz	0.07	120
meat	2½ oz	0.07	110
turkey	2½ oz	0.07	120
Health Valley			
brown rice cereal	½ oz or 2 T	1.34	110
sprouted cereal	½ oz or 2 T	4.2	110

❏ JAMS & JELLIES *See* FRUIT SPREADS

❏ JUICES & JUICE DRINKS
See BEVERAGES

❏ LAMB, VEAL, & MISCELLANEOUS MEATS

Lamb, veal, & other meats contain no dietary fiber.

	Portion	Fiber (g)	Calories

❑ LEGUMES & LEGUME PRODUCTS

Beans

adzuki
boiled	½ c	2.32 •	147
canned, sweetened	½ c	2.28 •	351
yokan (sugar & bean confection)	1½ oz	0.19 •	36

black turtle soup
boiled	1 c	3.76 •	241
canned	½ c	1.42 •	109
black, boiled	½ c	1.75 •	113

broad
raw	½ c	2.23 •	256
boiled	½ c	0.81 •	93
canned, solids & liquids	½ c	0.54 •	91

cannellini See kidney, below

cranberry
boiled	½ c	0.88 •	120
canned, solids & liquids	½ c	1.20 •	108

fava See broad, above

French, boiled	½ c	1.20 •	111

garbanzo See chickpeas, under Peas & Lentils, below

great northern
boiled	½ c	2.62 •	104
canned, solids & liquids	½ c	2.98 •	150

green gram See mung, below

hyacinth, boiled	½ c	2.36 •	114

kidney
California red, boiled	½ c	2.06 •	109

red
boiled	½ c	2.48 •	112
canned, solids & liquids	½ c	1.19 •	108
royal red, boiled	½ c	2.04 •	108

all other types
boiled	½ c	2.48 •	112
canned, solids & liquids	½ c	1.24 •	104

lima
baby, boiled	½ c	3.27 •	115

Fiber figures marked with • refer to *crude* fiber. Unmarked fiber figures refer to *dietary* fiber.

	Portion	Fiber (g)	Calories
lima *(cont.)*			
large			
boiled	½ c	2.90 •	108
canned, solids & liquids	½ c	1.48 •	95
frozen, boiled, drained	10 oz pkg	5.82 •	312
	½ c	1.59 •	85
long rice *See* mung, *below*			
lupins, boiled	½ c	0.55 •	98
miso *See* fermented products, *under* SOYBEANS & SOYBEAN PRODUCTS			
moth, boiled	½ c	1.19 •	103
mung			
boiled	½ c	0.46 •	107
long rice, dehydrated, prepared from mung bean starch	½ c	0.04 •	246
mature seeds, sprouted			
raw	12 oz pkg	2.77 •	102
	½ c	0.42 •	16
boiled, drained	½ c	0.32 •	13
canned, drained	½ c	0.16 •	8
stir-fried	½ c	0.43 •	31
mungo, boiled	½ c	1.20 •	95
natto *See* fermented products, *under* SOYBEANS & SOYBEAN PRODUCTS			
navy, canned, solids & liquids	½ c	2.44 •	148
okara *See* tofu: okara, *under* SOYBEANS & SOYBEAN PRODUCTS			
pink, boiled	½ c	1.34 •	125
pinto			
boiled	½ c	2.56 •	117
canned, solids & liquids	½ c	1.51 •	93
Roman *See* cranberry, *above*			
shellie *See* beans, shellie, *under* VEGETABLES, PLAIN & PREPARED			
small white, boiled	½ c	2.16 •	127
snap *See* beans, snap, *under* VEGETABLES, PLAIN & PREPARED			
soybeans *See* SOYBEANS & SOYBEAN PRODUCTS			
tempeh *See* fermented products, *under* SOYBEANS & SOYBEAN PRODUCTS			
white			
boiled	½ c	2.24 •	125
canned, solids & liquids	½ c	0.90 •	153
winged			
raw	½ c	6.23 •	372
boiled	½ c	2.11 •	126
winged bean leaves, raw	3½ oz	2.50 •	74
winged bean tuber, raw	3½ oz	7.40 •	159
yardlong			
raw	½ c	4.01 •	292
boiled	½ c	1.40 •	102

	Portion	Fiber (g)	Calories
yellow, boiled	½ c	1.00 •	126
yokan *See* adzuki, *above*			

Peas & Lentils

Bengal gram *See* chickpeas, *below*
black-eyed peas *See* cowpeas, common, *below*

	Portion	Fiber (g)	Calories
chickpeas			
boiled	½ c	2.05 •	134
canned, solids & liquids	½ c	1.63 •	143
cowpeas, catjang, boiled	½ c	1.36 •	100
cowpeas, common			
boiled	½ c	1.98 •	100
canned, plain, solids & liquids	½ c	0.81 •	92
frozen, boiled, drained	½ c	1.29 •	112
cowpeas, leafy tips			
raw	1 c	0.47 •	10
boiled, drained	½ c	0.68 •	6
cowpeas, young pods w/seeds			
raw	1 pod = 0.4 oz	0.20 •	5
boiled, drained	½ c	0.80 •	16
crowder peas *See* cowpeas, common, *above*			
golden gram *See* chickpeas, *above*			
lentils			
boiled	½ c	2.73 •	115
sprouted			
raw	½ c	1.16 •	40
stir-fried	3½ oz	1.10 •	101
pigeon peas			
raw	½ c	3.18 •	350
boiled	½ c	0.92 •	102
red gram *See* pigeon peas, *above*			
southern peas *See* cowpeas, common, *above*			
split peas, boiled	½ c	1.93 •	116

Prepared Bean Dishes

	Portion	Fiber (g)	Calories
baked beans			
canned			
plain or vegetarian	½ c	1.45 •	118

Fiber figures marked with • refer to *crude* fiber. Unmarked fiber figures refer to *dietary* fiber.

	Portion	Fiber (g)	Calories
baked beans: canned *(cont.)*			
w/franks	½ c	1.22 •	182
w/beef	½ c	1.40 •	161
w/pork	½ c	1.50 •	133
w/pork & sweet sauce	½ c	2.15 •	140
w/pork & tomato sauce	½ c	1.49 •	123
homemade	½ c	0.92 •	190
chili w/beans, canned	½ c	2.75 •	144
cowpeas, common, canned, w/pork	½ c	0.82 •	99
falafel	0.6 oz	0.18 •	57
	1.8 oz	0.55 •	170
hummus	1 c	3.33 •	420
refried beans, canned	½ c	4.00 •	134

■ BRAND NAME

Arrowhead Mills
anasazi beans	2 oz	12.01	200
chickpeas	2 oz	6.98	200
kidney beans	2 oz	11.75	190
lentils, green	2 oz	8.86	190
pinto beans	2 oz	11.18	200
split peas, green	2 oz	7.55	200

Fearn
lentil minestrone soup	½ of 3¾ oz box	7	160

Health Valley
BEANS
Boston baked, regular or no salt	4 oz	5.2	125
vegetarian, w/miso	4 oz	6.53	110

CHILI
con carne	4 oz	10.8	155
mild vegetarian w/beans, regular or no salt	4 oz	8.2	145
spicy vegetarian w/beans, regular or no salt	4 oz	8.2	145
w/lentils			
regular	4 oz	5.4	130
low-sodium	4 oz	4.6	142

	Portion	Fiber (g)	Calories
LENTILS			
Zesty pilaf, regular or no salt	4 oz	2.38	127
Joan of Arc Canned Vegetables			
blackeye peas	½ c	3.6	90
butter beans	½ c	3.7	80
Caliente Style chili beans	½ c	7.3	100
garbanzo beans	½ c	5.2	90
great northern beans	½ c	5.6	80
kidney beans, dark or light red	½ c	5.9	90
pinto beans	½ c	5.2	90
pork & beans in tomato sauce	½ c	5.2	90
Van Camp's			
Beanee Weenee	1 c	2.7 •	326
brown sugar beans	1 c	3.2 •	284
butter beans	1 c	2.8 •	162
chili			
w/beans	1 c	2.3 •	352
w/out beans	1 c	1.6 •	412
kidney beans			
dark red	1 c	2.3 •	182
light red	1 c	2.2 •	184
New Orleans–style red	1 c	2.4 •	178
Mexican-style chili beans	1 c	2.6 •	210
pork & beans	1 c	2.4 •	216
red beans	1 c	2.4 •	194
vegetarian-style beans	1 c	2.4 •	206
Western-style beans	1 c	2.4 •	207
Wolf			
chili			
w/beans	1 c	2.3 •	345
w/out beans			
regular	1 c	2 •	387
extra spicy	scant c	1.9 •	363

❑ **LUNCHEON MEATS** *See* PROCESSED
MEAT & POULTRY PRODUCTS

Fiber figures marked with • refer to *crude* fiber. Unmarked fiber figures refer
to *dietary* fiber.

	Portion	Fiber (g)	Calories

❑ **MAIN COURSES** *See* ENTREES & MAIN
COURSES, CANNED

❑ **MARMALADE** *See* FRUIT SPREADS

❑ **MAYONNAISE** *See* SALAD DRESSINGS
& MAYONNAISE

❑ **MEAT**

Meat contains no dietary fiber.

❑ **MEAT PRODUCTS, SIMULATED**
See NUTS & NUT-BASED BUTTERS,
FLOURS, MEALS, MILKS, PASTES,
& POWDERS

❑ **MILK, MILK SUBSTITUTES, & MILK
PRODUCTS**
See also Flavored Milk Beverages, *under*
BEVERAGES; CHEESE & CHEESE FOODS

Dairy products contain no dietary fiber. Fiber may be introduced in other
ingredients during preparation, as indicated in the following.

Yogurt

	Portion	Fiber (g)	Calories
fruit varieties, low-fat			
9 g protein	1 c	0.27 •	225
10 g protein	1 c	0.27 •	231
11 g protein	1 c	0.27 •	239

	Portion	Fiber (g)	Calories

Cream & Sour Cream Substitutes

coffee whitener, nondairy

liquid, frozen, containing hy-drogenated vegetable oil & soy protein	½ fl oz ½ c	0 • 0 •	20 163
liquid, frozen, containing lauric acid oil & sodium caseinate	½ fl oz ½ c	0 • 0 •	20 164
powdered, containing lauric acid oil & sodium caseinate	1 t	0 •	11
imitation sour cream, nondairy, cultured, containing lauric acid oil & sodium caseinate	1 oz 1 c	0 • 0 •	59 479
sour dressing, nonbutterfat, cultured (made by combin-ing fats or oils other than milk fat w/milk solids)	1 T 1 c	0 • 0 •	21 417

Milk Substitutes

filled (made by blending hy-drogenated vegetable oils w/milk solids)	1 c	0 •	154
filled, w/lauric acid oil (made by combining milk solids w/fats or oils other than milk fat)	1 c	0 •	153
imitation, containing blend of hydrogenated vegetable oils	1 c	0 •	150
imitation, containing lauric acid	1 c	0 •	150

❑ **MOLASSES** *See* SUGARS & SWEETENERS

Fiber figures marked with • refer to *crude* fiber. Unmarked fiber figures refer to *dietary* fiber.

	Portion	Fiber (g)	Calories

□ **MUFFINS** *See* **BREADS, ROLLS, BISCUITS, & MUFFINS**

□ **NOODLES & PASTA, PLAIN**

■ **BRAND NAME**

Health Valley
elbows

	Portion	Fiber (g)	Calories
whole-wheat	2 oz dry	7.15	197
whole-wheat w/4 vegetables	2 oz dry	7.66	197
lasagna, whole-wheat	2 oz dry	7.15	205
spaghetti			
whole-wheat	2 oz dry	7.15	205
whole-wheat w/amaranth	2 oz dry	8.8	197
whole-wheat w/spinach	2 oz dry	7.15	170
spinach lasagna, whole-wheat	2 oz dry	7.15	200

□ **NUTS & NUT-BASED BUTTERS, FLOURS, MEALS, MILKS, PASTES, & POWDERS**
See also SEEDS & SEED-BASED BUTTERS, FLOURS, & MEALS

	Portion	Fiber (g)	Calories
acorn flour, full-fat	1 oz	0.80 •	142
acorns			
raw	1 oz	0.73 •	105
dried	1 oz	0.96 •	145
almond butter			
plain	1 T	0.24 •	101
honey & cinnamon	1 T	0.24 •	96
almond meal, partially defatted	1 oz	0.65 •	116
almond paste	1 oz	1.70 •	127
	1 c firmly packed	13.62 •	1,012
almond powder			
full-fat	1 oz	0.54 •	168
	1 c not packed	1.24 •	385

	Portion	Fiber (g)	Calories
partially defatted	1 oz	0.80 •	112
	1 c not packed	1.82 •	255
almonds			
dried			
blanched	1 oz	0.65 •	166
	1 c whole kernels	3.32 •	850
unblanched	1 oz	0.77 •	167
	1 c whole kernels	3.85 •	837
dry-roasted, unblanched	1 oz	1.40 •	167
	1 c whole kernels	6.81 •	810
oil-roasted			
blanched	1 oz	0.89 •	174
	1 c whole kernels	4.43 •	870
unblanched	1 oz	1.40 •	176
	1 c whole kernels	7.74 •	970
toasted, unblanched	1 oz	1.41 •	167
beechnuts, dried	1 oz	1.05 •	164
Brazil nuts, dried, unblanched	1 oz	0.65 •	186
	1 c	3.20 •	919
butternuts, dried	1 oz	0.53 •	174
cashew butter, plain	1 T	0.12 •	94
cashew nuts			
dry-roasted	1 oz	0.20 •	163
	1 c wholes & halves	0.96 •	787
oil-roasted	1 oz	0.36 •	163
	1 c wholes & halves	1.65 •	748
chestnuts, Chinese			
raw	1 oz	0.47 •	64
boiled, steamed	1 oz	0.32 •	44
dried	1 oz	0.76 •	103
roasted	1 oz	0.50 •	68

Fiber figures marked with • refer to *crude* fiber. Unmarked fiber figures refer to *dietary* fiber.

	Portion	Fiber (g)	Calories
chestnuts, European			
raw			
unpeeled	1 oz	0.48 •	60
	1 c	2.48 •	308
peeled	1 oz	0.27 •	56
boiled, steamed	1 oz	0.20 •	37
dried			
unpeeled	1 oz	1.55 •	106
peeled	1 oz	1.42 •	105
roasted	1 oz	0.54 •	70
	1 c	2.72 •	350
chestnuts, Japanese			
raw	1 oz	0.28 •	44
boiled, steamed	1 oz	0.10 •	16
dried	1 oz	0.64 •	102
	1 c	3.51 •	558
roasted	1 oz	0.31 •	57
coconut meat			
raw	1.6 oz	1.92 •	159
	1 c shredded or grated	3.41 •	283
dried (desiccated)			
creamed	1 oz	1.12 •	194
sweetened, flaked, canned	4 oz	2.44 •	505
	1 c	1.65 •	341
sweetened, flaked, packaged	7 oz	4.17 •	944
	1 c	1.55 •	351
sweetened, shredded	7 oz	4.33 •	997
	1 c	2.02 •	466
toasted	1 oz	0.68 •	168
unsweetened	1 oz	1.51 •	187
coconut water	1 T	0.00 •	3
	1 c	0.05 •	46
filberts or hazelnuts			
dried			
blanched	1 oz	0.51 •	191
unblanched	1 oz	1.08 •	179
	1 c chopped kernels	4.37 •	727
dry-roasted, unblanched	1 oz	1.12 •	188
oil-roasted, unblanched	1 oz	0.71 •	187
formulated nuts, wheat-based			
macadamia-flavored	1 oz	0.17 •	176
unflavored	1 oz	0.23 •	177
all other flavors	1 oz	0.28 •	184

	Portion	Fiber (g)	Calories
ginkgo nuts			
raw	1 oz	0.14 •	52
canned	1 oz	0.46 •	32
	1 c	2.51 •	173
dried	1 oz	0.28 •	99
hazelnuts See filberts, above			
hickory nuts, dried	1 oz	0.92 •	187
macadamia nuts			
dried	1 oz	1.50 •	199
	1 c	7.08 •	940
oil-roasted	1 oz	0.49 •	204
	1 c wholes or halves	2.32 •	962
mixed nuts (cashew nuts, almonds, filberts, & pecans)			
dry-roasted, w/peanuts	1 oz	0.26 •	169
	1 c	1.23 •	814
oil-roasted			
w/peanuts	1 oz	0.61 •	175
	1 c	3.06 •	876
w/out peanuts	1 oz	0.63 •	175
	1 c	3.18 •	886
peanut butter, w/added fat, sugar, & salt			
chunk style	2 T	0.80 •	188
smooth style	2 T	0.77 •	188
peanut flour			
defatted	1 T	0.16 •	13
	1 c	2.43 •	196
peanuts			
Spanish, oil-roasted	1 oz	1.43 •	162
	1 c	7.49 •	851
Valencia, oil-roasted	1 oz	0.63 •	165
	1 c	3.25 •	848
Virginia, oil-roasted	1 oz	1.51 •	161
	1 c	7.69 •	826
other types			
raw	1 oz	1.36 •	159
	1 c	7.08 •	828
boiled	½ c	0.63 •	102

Fiber figures marked with • refer to *crude* fiber. Unmarked fiber figures refer to *dietary* fiber.

	Portion	Fiber (g)	Calories
peanuts, other types *(cont.)*			
dry-roasted	1 oz	1.43 •	164
	1 c	7.45 •	855
oil-roasted	1 oz	1.49 •	163
	1 c	7.68 •	837
pecan flour	1 oz	0.43 •	93
pecans			
dried	1 oz	0.45 •	190
	1 c halves	1.72 •	721
dry-roasted	1 oz	0.47 •	187
oil-roasted	1 oz	0.46 •	195
	1 c	1.77 •	754
pignolias *See* pine nuts, *below*			
pili nuts, dried	1 oz	0.80 •	204
	1 c	3.36 •	863
pine nuts			
pignolia, dried	1 T	0.08 •	51
	1 oz	0.23 •	146
piñon, dried	10 kernels	0.05 •	6
	1 oz	1.34 •	161
pistachios			
dried	1 oz	0.53 •	164
	1 c	2.40 •	739
dry-roasted	1 oz	0.51 •	172
	1 c	2.31 •	776
sweet chestnuts *See* chestnuts, European, *above*			
walnuts			
black, dried	1 oz	1.83 •	172
	1 c chopped	8.08 •	759
English or Persian, dried	1 oz	1.31 •	182
	1 c pieces	5.52 •	770

▪ BRAND NAME

Blue Diamond
almonds			
raw, whole, unblanched	1 oz	0.68 •	173
blanched, whole, raw	1 oz	0.57 •	174
blanched, sliced	1 oz	0.50 •	176
dry-roasted, unsalted	1 oz	0.7 •	168
oil-roasted, salted	1 oz	0.9 •	174
hazelnuts			
raw, whole, Oregon	1 oz	0.7 •	166

	Portion	Fiber (g)	Calories
oil-roasted, salted	1 oz	0.7 •	180
macadamia nuts, dry-roasted, salted	1 oz	0.5 •	193
pistachios, dry-roasted, salted, natural, California	1 oz	0.7 •	162
Fearn			
Brazil nut burger mix	¼ c dry or ⅛ of 7.6 oz box	4.1	100
Skippy Peanut Butter			
creamy	1 T	0.3 •	95
	2 T	0.6 •	190
Super Chunk	1 T	0.3 •	95
	2 T	0.6 •	190

❑ **OILS** *See* FATS, OILS, & SHORTENINGS

❑ **PASTA** *See* NOODLES & PASTA, PLAIN

❑ **PASTRIES** *See* DESSERTS: CAKES, PASTRIES, & PIES

❑ **PÂTÉS** *See* PROCESSED MEAT & POULTRY PRODUCTS

❑ **PEANUT BUTTER** *See* NUTS & NUT-BASED BUTTERS, FLOURS, MEALS, MILKS, PASTES, & POWDERS

Fiber figures marked with • refer to *crude* fiber. Unmarked fiber figures refer to *dietary* fiber.

	Portion	Fiber (g)	Calories

❑ PICKLES & RELISHES
See also peppers *under* VEGETABLES, PLAIN
& PREPARED

PICKLES, CUCUMBER
bread & butter	4 slices	0.1 •	18
sour	1 large	0.5 •	10
sweet	1 large	0.5 •	146

RELISHES
chow chow			
sour	1 oz	0.2 •	8
sweet	1 oz	0.3 •	32

❑ PIES *See* DESSERTS: CAKES, PASTRIES, & PIES

❑ PIZZA

▪ BRAND NAME

Celeste Frozen Pizza
Canadian-style bacon	7¾ oz pizza	0.7 •	541
	¼ of 19 oz pizza	0.5 •	329
cheese	6½ oz pizza	0.7 •	497
	¼ of 17¾ oz pizza	0.5 •	317
deluxe	8¼ oz pizza	1.2 •	582
	¼ of 22¼ oz pizza	0.8 •	378
pepperoni	6¾ oz pizza	0.8 •	546
	¼ of 19 oz pizza	0.5 •	368
sausage	7½ oz pizza	1.1 •	571
	¼ of 20 oz pizza	0.7 •	376
sausage & mushroom	8½ oz pizza	1.2 •	592
	¼ of 22½ oz pizza	1.0 •	387

	Portion	Fiber (g)	Calories
Suprema	9 oz pizza	1.3 •	678
	¼ of 23 oz pizza	0.8 •	381

◻ PORK, FRESH & CURED

Fresh & cured pork & pork variety meats contain no dietary fiber.

◻ POULTRY, FRESH & PROCESSED

Meat & organs from domesticated & wild fowl contains no dietary fiber. Fiber may be introduced in other ingredients during preparation, as indicated in the following.

Chicken, Broilers or Fryers

Values are based on a chicken weighing 3.33 lbs as purchased with giblets & neck.

	Portion	Fiber (g)	Calories
flesh, skin, giblets, & neck, fried			
batter-dipped	1 chicken	0.36 •	2,987
flour-coated	1 chicken	0.09 •	1,928
flesh & skin, fried			
batter-dipped	½ chicken	0.17 •	1,347
flour-coated	½ chicken	0.04 •	844
flesh only, fried	1 c	0.01 •	307
skin only, fried			
batter-dipped	½ chicken	0.17 •	748
flour-coated	½ chicken	0.02 •	281
giblets, fried, flour-coated	1 c	0.02 •	402
light meat w/skin, fried			
batter-dipped	½ chicken	0.07 •	520
flour-coated	½ chicken	0.01 •	320
dark meat w/skin, fried			
batter-dipped	½ chicken	0.10 •	828
flour-coated	½ chicken	0.03 •	523

Fiber figures marked with • refer to *crude* fiber. Unmarked fiber figures refer to *dietary* fiber.

	Portion	Fiber (g)	Calories
light meat w/out skin, fried	1 c	0.00 •	268
dark meat w/out skin, fried	1 c	0.01 •	334
back, meat & skin, fried			
batter-dipped	½ back	0.05 •	397
flour-coated	½ back	0.02 •	238
back, meat only, fried	½ back	0.01 •	167
breast, meat & skin, fried			
batter-dipped	½ breast	0.05 •	364
flour-coated	½ breast	0.01 •	218
breast, meat only, fried	½ breast	0.00 •	161
drumstick, meat & skin, fried			
batter-dipped	1	0.02 •	193
flour-coated	1	0.00 •	120
drumstick, meat only, fried	1	0.00 •	82
leg (drumstick & thigh), meat & skin, fried			
batter-dipped	1	0.05 •	431
flour-coated	1	0.01 •	285
leg (drumstick & thigh), meat only, fried	1	0.00 •	195
neck, meat & skin, fried			
batter-dipped	1	0.02 •	172
flour-coated	1	0.01 •	119
neck, meat only, fried	1	0.00 •	50
thigh, meat & skin, fried			
batter-dipped	1	0.03 •	238
flour-coated	1	0.01 •	162
thigh, meat only, fried	1	0.00 •	113
wing, meat & skin, fried			
batter-dipped	1	0.02 •	159
flour-coated	1	0.00 •	103
wing, meat only, fried	1	0.00 •	42
TURKEY, PROCESSED			
gravy & turkey, frozen	5 oz	0.42 •	95

❏ **POULTRY SPREADS** *See* PROCESSED MEAT & POULTRY PRODUCTS

❏ **PRESERVES** *See* FRUIT SPREADS

	Portion	Fiber (g)	Calories

❑ PROCESSED MEAT & POULTRY PRODUCTS

Meat & poultry sausages, frankfurters, cold cuts, tés, & spreads contain no dietary fiber.

❑ PUDDING DESSERTS, FROZEN
See DESSERTS, FROZEN

❑ PUDDINGS *See* DESSERTS: CUSTARDS, GELATINS, & PUDDINGS

❑ RELISHES *See* PICKLES & RELISHES

❑ RICE & GRAINS, PLAIN & PREPARED
See also VEGETABLES, PLAIN & PREPARED

hominy grits *See* corn grits, *under* BREAKFAST CEREALS, COLD & HOT

■ BRAND NAME

Arrowhead Mills
PLAIN RICE & GRAINS

	Portion	Fiber (g)	Calories
barley, pearled	2 oz	7.2	200
bulgur wheat	2 oz	5.45	200
millet	2 oz	1.84	90
oat groats	2 oz	5.56	220
quinoa	2 oz	5.33	200
rice, brown, long	2 oz	3.12	200

Fiber figures marked with • refer to *crude* fiber. Unmarked fiber figures refer to *dietary* fiber.

	Portion	Fiber (g)	Calories
wheat, hard, red, or winter	2 oz	8.34	190
PREPARED RICE & GRAINS			
quick brown rice			
regular	2 oz	0.30	200
Spanish style	¼ of 5.65 oz pkg	0.08	150
vegetable herb	¼ of 5.6 oz pkg	0.11	150
wild rice & herbs	¼ of 5.35 oz pkg	0.10	140
Fearn			
Naturfresh corn germ	¼ c or 1 oz	1.3 •	130
Health Valley			
amaranth pilaf			
regular	4 oz	8.21	210
no salt	4 oz	3.7	100
Pillsbury Frozen Rice Originals			
Italian blend white rice & spinach in cheese sauce	½ c	0.0 •	170
long grain white & wild rice	½ c	0.0 •	120
rice & broccoli in flavored cheese sauce	½ c	0.0 •	120
Rice Jubilee	½ c	0.0 •	150
Rice Medley	½ c	0.0 •	120
rice pilaf	½ c	0.0 •	120
rice w/herb butter sauce	½ c	0.0 •	150
Quaker Oats			
Scotch brand pearled barley, medium or quick	¼ c	0.4 •	172
Van Camp's			
Golden Hominy	1 c	0.8 •	128
Spanish rice	1 c	0.6 •	150

❏ **ROLLS** *See* BREADS, ROLLS, BISCUITS, & MUFFINS

	Portion	Fiber (g)	Calories

❑ SALAD DRESSINGS & MAYONNAISE

Mayonnaise

Mayonnaise contains no dietary fiber.

Salad Dressings

	Portion	Fiber (g)	Calories
bleu cheese, commercial			
regular	1 c	0.2 •	1,235
	1 T	0.0 •	77
low-cal	1 T	tr •	11
cooked, homemade	1 c	0.0 •	400
	1 T	0.0 •	25
French			
commercial			
regular	1 c	1.9 •	1,074
	1 T	0.1 •	67
creamy	1 T	1.0 •	70
low-cal	1 c	0.7 •	349
	1 T	0.0 •	22
homemade	1 c	0.4 •	1,388
	1 T	0.0 •	88
Italian, commercial			
regular	1 c	0.5 •	1,098
	1 T	0.0 •	69
low-cal	1 c	0.7 •	253
	1 T	0.0 •	16
Russian, commercial			
regular	1 c	0.7 •	1,210
	1 T	0.0 •	76
low-cal	1 c	0.9 •	368
	1 T	0.1 •	23
sesame seed, commercial	1 c	0.9 •	1,086
	1 T	0.1 •	68
Thousand Island, commercial			
regular	1 c	5.0 •	943
	1 T	0.3 •	59
low-cal	1 c	2.9 •	389
	1 T	0.2 •	24

Fiber figures marked with • refer to *crude* fiber. Unmarked fiber figures refer to *dietary* fiber.

	Portion	Fiber (g)	Calories

□ SAUCES & GRAVIES

Gravies

	Portion	Fiber (g)	Calories
au jus			
dehydrated, prepared w/water	1 c	0.01 •	19
	21.7 oz	0.03 •	48
brown, dehydrated, prepared	1 c	0.01 •	9
w/water	9.7 oz	0.01 •	9
chicken, dehydrated, prepared w/water	1 c	0.06 •	83
turkey, dehydrated, prepared w/water	1 c	0.10 •	87

Sauces

	Portion	Fiber (g)	Calories
barbecue, ready-to-serve	1 c	1.50 •	188
béarnaise			
dehydrated	0.9 oz	0.05 •	90
dehydrated, prepared w/milk	1 c	0.03 •	701
& butter	13½ oz	0.05 •	1,052
cheese			
dehydrated	1.2 oz	0.04 •	158
dehydrated, prepared w/whole milk	1 c	0.04 •	307
curry			
dehydrated	1.2 oz	0.46 •	151
dehydrated, prepared w/whole milk	1 c	0.37 •	270
	12 oz	0.46 •	337
hollandaise, dehydrated			
w/butterfat	1.2 oz	0.03 •	187
w/butterfat, prepared w/water	1 c	0.04 •	237
	7.2 oz	0.03 •	187
w/vegetable oil	1 oz	0.05 •	93
w/vegetable oil, prepared	1 c	0.03 •	703
w/milk & butter	13½ oz	0.05 •	1,055
marinara, canned	1 c	1.65 •	171
	15½ oz	2.90 •	300
mushroom			
dehydrated	1 oz	0.28 •	99
dehydrated, prepared w/whole milk	1 c	0.23 •	228
	11.7 oz	0.28 •	285

	Portion	Fiber (g)	Calories
spaghetti			
canned	1 c	2.33 •	272
	15½ oz	4.10 •	479
Stroganoff			
dehydrated	1.6 oz	0.60 •	161
dehydrated, prepared w/whole	1 c	0.56 •	271
milk & water	11.2 oz	0.06 •	292
tomato paste & puree *See* VEGETABLES, PLAIN & PREPARED			
tomato, canned	½ c	0.87 •	37
w/mushrooms	½ c	1.03 •	42
w/onions	½ c	0.98 •	52
w/tomato tidbits	½ c	1.34 •	39
white			
dehydrated	1.7 oz	0.10 •	230
dehydrated, prepared w/whole	1 c	0.04 •	241
milk	23.2 oz	0.10 •	602

- **BRAND NAME**

Wolf

chili hot dog sauce	about ⅙ c	0.4 •	44

❑ SEAFOOD & SEAFOOD PRODUCTS

Finfish & shellfish contain no dietary fiber. Fiber may be introduced in other ingredients during preparation, as indicated in the following.

Finfish

catfish, channel, breaded & fried	3 oz	0.36 •	194
croaker, Atlantic, breaded & fried	3 oz	0.12 •	188

Fiber figures marked with • refer to *crude* fiber. Unmarked fiber figures refer to *dietary* fiber.

	Portion	Fiber (g)	Calories
shark, mixed species, batter-dipped & fried	3 oz	0.150 •	194

Seafood Products

	Portion	Fiber (g)	Calories
crab cakes (blue crab)	2.1 oz	0.03 •	93
fish sticks (walleye pollock), frozen, reheated	1 stick = 1 oz	0.12 •	76
gefilte fish, commercial, sweet recipe w/broth	1½ oz	0.02 •	35
tuna salad	3 oz	0.46 •	159
	1 c	1.11 •	383

Shellfish

	Portion	Fiber (g)	Calories
abalone, mixed species, fried	3 oz	0.11 •	161
clams, mixed species			
breaded & fried	20 small (110/qt)	0.28 •	379
	3 oz	0.13 •	171
oysters, eastern			
breaded & fried	6 medium (70/qt)	0.13 •	173
	3 oz	0.13 •	167
scallops, mixed species, breaded & fried	2 large (30/lb)	0.05 •	67
shrimp, mixed species			
breaded & fried	4 large (32/lb)	0.04 •	73
	3 oz	0.12 •	206
squid, mixed species, fried	3 oz	0.11 •	149

❑ SEASONINGS

See also BREADCRUMBS, CROUTONS, STUFFINGS, & SEASONED COATINGS; SAUCES & GRAVIES; VEGETABLES, PLAIN & PREPARED

	Portion	Fiber (g)	Calories
allspice, ground	1 t	0.41 •	5
anise seed	1 t	0.31 •	7
basil, ground	1 t	0.25 •	4
bay leaf, crumbled	1 t	0.16 •	2
caraway seed	1 t	0.27 •	7
cardamon, ground	1 t	0.23 •	6
celery seed	1 t	0.24 •	8

	Portion	Fiber (g)	Calories
chervil, dried	1 t	0.07 •	1
chili pepper	1 t	0.3 •	9
chili powder	1 t	0.58 •	8
cinnamon, ground	1 t	0.56 •	6
cloves, ground	1 t	0.20 •	7
coriander leaf, dried	1 t	0.06 •	2
coriander seed	1 t	0.52 •	5
cumin seed	1 t	0.22 •	8
curry powder	1 t	0.33 •	6
dill seed	1 t	0.44 •	6
dillweed, dried	1 t	0.12 •	3
fennel seed	1 t	0.31 •	7
fenugreek seed	1 t	0.37 •	12
garlic powder	1 t	0.05 •	9
ginger, ground	1 t	0.11 •	6
mace, ground	1 t	0.08 •	8
marjoram, dried	1 t	0.11 •	2
mustard powder	1 t	tr •	9
mustard seed, yellow	1 t	0.22 •	15
nutmeg, ground	1 t	0.09 •	12
onion powder	1 t	0.12 •	7
oregano, ground	1 t	0.22 •	5
paprika	1 t	0.44 •	6
parsley, dried	1 t	0.03 •	4
pepper, black	1 t	0.28 •	5
pepper, red/cayenne	1 t	0.45 •	6
pepper, seasoned	1 t	0.2 •	10
pepper, white	1 t	0.10 •	7
poppy seed	1 t	0.18 •	15
poultry seasoning	1 t	0.17 •	5
pumpkin pie spice	1 t	0.25 •	6
rosemary, dried	1 t	0.21 •	4
saffron	1 t	0.03 •	2
sage, ground	1 t	0.13 •	2
salt	1 t	0.0 •	0
savory, ground	1 t	0.21 •	4
tarragon, ground	1 t	0.12 •	5

Fiber figures marked with • refer to *crude* fiber. Unmarked fiber figures refer to *dietary* fiber.

	Portion	Fiber (g)	Calories
thyme, ground	1 t	0.26 •	4
tumeric, ground	1 t	0.15 •	8

▪ BRAND NAME

Lawry's

onion salt	1 t	0.1 •	7
seasoning salt	1 t	tr •	3

Morton

lite salt	1 t	0.0 •	0
salt substitute	1 t	0.0 •	0

❑ SEEDS & SEED-BASED BUTTERS, FLOURS, & MEALS

See also NUTS & NUT-BASED BUTTERS, FLOURS, MEALS, MILKS, PASTES, & POWDERS

alfalfa seeds, sprouted, raw	1 c	0.54 •	10
breadfruit seeds			
raw	1 oz	0.48 •	54
boiled	1 oz	0.51 •	48
roasted	1 oz	0.62 •	59
breadnuttree seeds			
raw	1 oz	0.72 •	62
dried	1 oz	1.59 •	104
chia seeds, dried	1 oz	7.19 •	134
cottonseed flour			
partially defatted	1 T	0.10 •	18
	1 c	1.88 •	337
low-fat	1 oz	0.69 •	94
cottonseed kernels, roasted	1 T	0.20 •	51
	1 c	2.98 •	754
cottonseed meal, partially defatted	1 oz	0.69 •	104
lotus seeds			
raw	1 oz	0.18 •	25
dried	1 oz	0.69 •	94
	1 c	0.77 •	106
pumpkin & squash seeds			
whole, roasted	1 oz	10.20 •	127
	1 c	22.98 •	285

	Portion	Fiber (g)	Calories
kernels			
dried	1 oz	0.63 •	154
	1 c	3.07 •	747
roasted	1 oz	0.51 •	148
	1 c	4.11 •	1,184
ramons *See* breadnuttree seeds, *above*			
safflower seed kernels, dried	1 oz	0.70 •	147
safflower seed meal, partially defatted	1 oz	2.16 •	97
sesame butter			
paste	1 oz	1.55 •	169
	1 T	0.87 •	95
tahini			
from raw & stone-ground	1 oz	1.42 •	162
kernels	1 T	0.75 •	86
from roasted & toasted	1 oz	1.42 •	169
kernels	1 T	0.75 •	89
from unroasted kernels	1 oz	0.86 •	173
	1 T	0.42 •	85
sesame flour			
high-fat	1 oz	1.81 •	149
partially defatted	1 oz	1.71 •	109
low-fat	1 oz	1.42 •	95
sesame meal, partially defatted	1 oz	1.14 •	161
sesame seeds			
whole			
dried	1 c	6.62 •	825
roasted & toasted	1 oz	2.41 •	161
kernels			
dried	1 T	0.24 •	47
	1 c	4.44 •	882
toasted	1 oz	1.42 •	161
	1 T	0.41 •	52
sisymbrium sp. seeds, whole, dried	1 oz	8.43 •	90
	1 c	21.98 •	235
squash seeds *See* pumpkin & squash seeds, *above*			
sunflower seed butter	1 T	0.24 •	93
sunflower seed flour, partially defatted	1 T	0.26 •	16
	1 c	4.15 •	261

Fiber figures marked with • refer to *crude* fiber. Unmarked fiber figures refer to *dietary* fiber.

	Portion	Fiber (g)	Calories
sunflower seed kernels			
dried	1 oz	1.18 •	162
	1 c	5.99 •	821
dry-roasted	1 oz	0.51 •	165
	1 c	2.32 •	745
oil-roasted	1 oz	0.51 •	175
	1 c	2.41 •	830
toasted	1 oz	0.52 •	176
	1 c	2.43 •	829
tahini *See* sesame butter: tahini, *above*			
watermelon seed kernels, dried	1 oz	0.86 •	158
	1 c	3.29 •	602

▪ BRAND NAME

Arrowhead Mills
amaranth seeds	2 oz	1.95	200
flax seeds	1 oz	5.99	140
sesame seeds, hulled	1 oz	3.66	160
sesame tahini, chemical-free	1 oz	2.64	170
sunflower seeds, hulled	1 oz	2.21	160

❑ SHORTENINGS *See* FATS, OILS, & SHORTENINGS

❑ SNACKS
See also CRACKERS

cheese puffs	1 oz	0.2 •	159
cheese straws	4	tr •	109

▪ BRAND NAME

Cornnuts
original flavor	1 oz	2.66	120
barbecue flavor	1 oz	2.51	110
nacho cheese flavor	1 oz	2.38	110
unsalted	1 oz	2.66	120

	Portion	Fiber (g)	Calories
Health Valley			
CORN CHIPS			
regular or no salt	1 oz	1.0	163
POTATO CHIPS			
Country Chips, regular or no salt	1 oz	0.9	160
Country Ripples, regular or no salt	1 oz	0.9	160
dip, regular, or no salt	1 oz	0.9	160
SNACK PUFFS			
Carrot Lites	1 oz	0.92	74
Cheddar Lites, w/green onion or no salt	1 oz	0.24	60
TORTILLA CHIPS			
Buenitos			
regular or no salt	1 oz	3.6	152
nacho cheese & chili	1 oz	0.48	150

❑ SOUPS, PREPARED

Canned

	Portion	Fiber (g)	Calories
asparagus, cream of, condensed	1 can = 10¾ oz	1.83 •	210
prepared w/water	1 c	0.73 •	87
prepared w/whole milk	1 c	0.74 •	161
	1 can	1.81 •	392
bean, black, condensed, prepared w/water	1 c	1.31 •	116
bean w/bacon, condensed	1 can = 11½ oz	4.24 •	420
prepared w/water	1 c	1.52 •	173
bean w/frankfurter, condensed	1 can = 11¼ oz	4.15 •	454
prepared w/water	1 c	1.50 •	187

Fiber figures marked with • refer to *crude* fiber. Unmarked fiber figures refer to *dietary* fiber.

	Portion	Fiber (g)	Calories
beef broth or bouillon, ready-to-serve	1 c	tr •	16
	1 can = 14 oz	tr •	27
beef noodle, condensed	1 can = 10¾ oz	0.31 •	204
prepared w/water	1 c	tr •	84
beef, chunky, ready-to-serve	1 c	0.72 •	171
	1 can = 19 oz	1.62 •	383
celery, cream of, condensed	1 can = 10¾ oz	0.92 •	219
prepared w/water	1 c	0.38 •	90
prepared w/whole milk	1 c	0.38 •	165
	1 can	0.92 •	400
chicken broth, condensed	1 can = 10¾ oz	tr •	94
prepared w/water	1 c	tr •	39
chicken gumbo, condensed	1 can = 10¾ oz	0.61 •	137
prepared w/water	1 c	0.24 •	56
chicken noodle, condensed	1 can = 10½ oz	0.30 •	182
prepared w/water	1 c	0.24 •	75
chicken noodle w/meatballs, ready-to-serve	1 c	0.55 •	99
	1 can = 20 oz	1.25 •	227
chicken rice, condensed	1 can = 10½ oz	0.30 •	146
prepared w/water	1 c	tr •	60
chicken vegetable, condensed	1 can = 10½ oz	0.30 •	181
prepared w/water	1 c	0.12 •	74
chicken, chunky, ready-to-serve	1 c	0.25 •	178
	1 can = 10¾ oz	0.31 •	216
chicken, cream of, condensed	1 can = 10¾ oz	0.31 •	283
prepared w/water	1 c	0.12 •	116
prepared w/whole milk	1 c	0.13 •	191
	1 can	0.31 •	464
chili beef, condensed	1 can = 11¼ oz	3.51 •	411
prepared w/water	1 c	1.45 •	169
clam chowder (Manhattan)			
chunky, ready-to-serve	1 c	0.48 •	133
	1 can = 19 oz	1.08 •	299

	Portion	Fiber (g)	Calories
condensed	1 can = 10¾ oz	0.92 •	187
condensed, prepared w/water	1 c	0.49 •	78
clam chowder (New England), condensed, prepared w/ water	1 c	0.27 •	95
crab, ready-to-serve	1 c	0.54 •	76
	1 can = 13 oz	0.81 •	114
escarole, ready-to-serve	1 c	0.74 •	27
	1 can = 19½ oz	1.66 •	61
gazpacho, ready-to-serve	1 c	0.78 •	57
	1 can = 13 oz	1.18 •	87
lentil w/ham, ready-to-serve	1 c	1.40 •	140
	1 can = 20 oz	3.20 •	320
minestrone, condensed	1 can = 10½ oz	1.79 •	202
prepared w/water	1 c	0.72 •	83
mushroom, cream of, condensed	1 can = 10¾ oz	0.61 •	313
prepared w/water	1 c	0.46 •	129
prepared w/whole milk	1 c	0.25 •	203
	1 can	0.61 •	494
onion, condensed	1 can = 10½ oz	1.19 •	138
prepared w/water	1 c	0.48 •	57
pea, green, condensed	1 can = 11¼ oz	1.60 •	398
prepared w/water	1 c	0.66 •	164
prepared w/whole milk	1 c	0.66 •	239
	1 can	1.60 •	579
pea, split, w/ham, condensed	1 can = 11½ oz	1.63 •	459
prepared w/water	1 c	0.67 •	189
pepperpot, condensed	1 can = 10½ oz	1.19 •	251
prepared w/water	1 c	0.48 •	103
stockpot, condensed	1 can = 11 oz	1.25 •	242
prepared w/water	1 c	0.49 •	100
tomato rice, condensed	1 can = 11 oz	1.56 •	291
prepared w/water	1 c	0.64 •	120

Fiber figures marked with • refer to *crude* fiber. Unmarked fiber figures refer to *dietary* fiber.

	Portion	Fiber (g)	Calories
tomato, condensed	1 can = 10¾ oz	1.22 •	208
prepared w/water	1 c	0.49 •	86
prepared w/whole milk	1 c	0.50 •	160
	1 can	1.20 •	389
turkey noodle, condensed	1 can = 10¾ oz	0.31 •	168
prepared w/water	1 c	0.24 •	69
turkey, chunky, ready-to-serve	1 c	0.94 •	136
	1 can = 18¾ oz	2.13 •	306
vegetable w/beef broth, condensed	1 can = ½ oz	1.49 •	197
prepared w/water	1 c	0.72 •	81
vegetable w/beef, condensed	1 can = 10¾ oz	0.76 •	192
prepared w/water	1 c	0.31 •	79
vegetable, chunky, ready-to-serve	1 c	1.20 •	122
	1 can = 19 oz	2.70 •	274
vegetable, vegetarian, condensed	1 can = ½ oz	1.19 •	176
prepared w/water	1 c	0.49 •	72

Dehydrated

	Portion	Fiber (g)	Calories
asparagus, cream of, prepared w/water	1 c	0.13 •	59
	39.7 oz	0.58 •	265
bean w/bacon, prepared w/water	1 c	1.53 •	105
beef broth or bouillon, prepared w/water	1 c	0.01 •	19
	6 fl oz	0.01 •	14
beef noodle, prepared w/water	1 c	0.06 •	41
	6 fl oz	0.04 •	30
cauliflower, prepared w/water	1 c	0.19 •	68
celery, cream of, prepared w/water	1 c	0.19 •	63
chicken broth or bouillon, prepared w/water	1 c	0.01 •	21
	6 fl oz	0.01 •	16
chicken noodle	1 pkt = 0.4 oz	0.05 •	38
	1 pkt = 2.6 oz	0.30 •	257

	Portion	Fiber (g)	Calories
prepared w/water	1 c	0.06 •	53
chicken, cream of, prepared	1 c	1.16 •	107
w/water	6 fl oz	0.87 •	80
clam chowder (Manhattan)	1 c	0.57 •	65
clam chowder (New England)	1 c	0.20 •	95
consommé, w/gelatin added,	1 c	0.01 •	17
prepared w/water	39½ oz	0.06 •	77
leek, prepared w/water	1 c	0.26 •	71
	36 fl oz	1.19 •	319
minestrone, prepared w/water	1 c	0.42 •	79
	40.2 oz	1.90 •	358
mushroom	1 pkt regular = 2.6 oz	0.25 •	328
	1 pkt instant = 0.6 oz	0.06 •	74
prepared w/water	1 c	0.07 •	96
onion	1 pkt = 1.4 oz	0.94 •	115
	1 pkt = ¼ oz	0.17 •	21
prepared w/water	1 c	0.23 •	28
oxtail, prepared w/water	1 c	0.13 •	71
	36 fl oz	0.59 •	318
pea, green or split	1 pkt = 4 oz	2.08 •	402
	1 pkt = 1 oz	0.52 •	100
prepared w/water	1 c	0.69 •	133
tomato (includes cream of tomato)	1 pkt = ¾ oz	0.32 •	77
prepared w/water	1 c	0.43 •	102
	6 fl oz	0.32 •	77
tomato vegetable (includes Italian vegetable & spring vegetable)	1 pkt = 1.4 oz	1.19 •	125
prepared w/water	1 c	0.53 •	55
	6 fl oz	0.40 •	41
vegetable beef, prepared	1 c	0.15 •	53
w/water	1 pkt = 40 oz	0.69 •	240

Fiber figures marked with • refer to *crude* fiber. Unmarked fiber figures refer to *dietary* fiber.

	Portion	Fiber (g)	Calories
vegetable, cream of, prepared	1 c	0.14 •	105
w/water	6 fl oz	0.11 •	79

• BRAND NAME

Health Valley

bean, regular or no salt	7½ oz	4.0	154
five bean, chunky, regular or no salt	7½ oz	4.98	100
clam chowder, regular or no salt	7½ oz	1.78	110
green split pea, regular or no salt	7½ oz	7.83	158
lentil, regular or no salt	7½ oz	4.38	163
minestrone, regular or no salt	7½ oz	5.8	115
mushroom barley			
no salt	7½ oz	2.63	110
regular	7½ oz	2.63	107
potato leek, regular or no salt	7½ oz	1.71	107
tomato, regular or no salt	7½ oz	0.385	100
vegetable, regular or no salt	7½ oz	6.8	100

❑ SOUR CREAM *See* MILK, MILK SUBSTITUTES, & MILK PRODUCTS

❑ SOYBEANS & SOYBEAN PRODUCTS

Soybean Products

fermented products			
miso	½ c	3.41 •	284
natto	½ c	1.41 •	187
tempeh	½ c	2.48 •	165
soy flour			
full-fat			
raw	½ c stirred	1.98 •	182
roasted	½ c stirred	0.93 •	184

	Portion	Fiber (g)	Calories
low-fat	½ c stirred	1.86 •	163
defatted	½ c stirred	2.14 •	164
soy meal, defatted, raw	½ c	3.53 •	206
soy protein			
concentrate	1 oz	1.05 •	92
isolate	1 oz	0.07 •	94
tofu			
dried-frozen (koyadofu)			
prepared w/calcium sulfate	0.6 oz	0.03 •	82
prepared w/nigari	0.6 oz	0.03 •	82
fried			
prepared w/calcium sulfate	½ oz	0.02 •	35
prepared w/nigari	½ oz	0.02 •	35
okara	½ c	2.51 •	47
raw			
regular, made w/calcium	4.1 oz	0.09 •	88
sulfate	½ c	0.09 •	94
regular, made w/nigari	4.1 oz	0.09 •	88
	½ c	0.09 •	94
firm, made w/calcium sulfate	2.9 oz	0.12 •	118
	½ c	0.18 •	183
firm, made w/nigari	2.9 oz	0.12 •	118
	½ c	0.18 •	183
salted & fermented (fuyu)			
prepared w/calcium sulfate	0.4 oz	0.03 •	13
prepared w/nigari	0.4 oz	0.03 •	13

Soybeans

	Portion	Fiber (g)	Calories
boiled	½ c	1.75 •	149
dry-roasted	½ c	4.63 •	387
mature seeds, sprouted, raw	½ c	0.8 •	46
roasted	½ c	3.96 •	405

• BRAND NAME

Arrowhead Mills

	Portion	Fiber (g)	Calories
soybeans	2 oz	13.23	230
Kikkoman			
stir-fry sauce	1 t	tr	6

Fiber figures marked with • refer to *crude* fiber. Unmarked fiber figures refer to *dietary* fiber.

	Portion	Fiber (g)	Calories

❑ **SPICES** *See* SEASONINGS

❑ **STUFFINGS** *See* BREADCRUMBS,
CROUTONS, STUFFINGS, & SEASONED
COATINGS

❑ **SUGARS & SWEETENERS**

Honey, molasses, sugar, syrup, & treacle contain no dietary fiber.

❑ **SYRUP** *See* SUGARS & SWEETENERS

❑ **TREACLE** *See* SUGARS & SWEETENERS

❑ **TURKEY** *See* POULTRY, FRESH
& PROCESSED

❑ **VEAL** *See* LAMB, VEAL,
& MISCELLANEOUS MEATS

❑ **VEGETABLES, PLAIN & PREPARED**
See also LEGUMES & LEGUME PRODUCTS; PICKLES
& RELISHES; RICE & GRAINS, PLAIN & PREPARED

Vegetables, Plain

	Portion	Fiber (g)	Calories
alfalfa seeds *See* SEEDS & SEED-BASED BUTTERS, FLOURS, & MEALS			
amaranth			
raw	1 c	0.27 •	7
boiled, drained	½ c	0.86 •	14

	Portion	Fiber (g)	Calories
arrowhead			
raw	1 medium corm = 0.4 oz	0.10 •	12
boiled, drained	1 medium corm = 1.4 oz	0.18 •	9
artichokes, globe & French varieties			
boiled	1 medium = 4.2 oz	39	53
	½ c hearts	39	37
frozen, boiled, drained	9 oz pkg	2.21 •	108
artichokes, Jerusalem See Jerusalem artichokes, *below*			
asparagus beans See yardlong beans, *under* LEGUMES & LEGUME PRODUCTS			
asparagus, cuts & spears			
raw	4 spears = 2 oz	0.48 •	13
boiled	4 spears = 2.1 oz	0.50 •	15
canned, solids & liquids	½ c	0.64 •	17
frozen, boiled, drained	4 spears = 2.1 oz	0.50 •	17
	10 oz pkg	2.45 •	82
balsam pear			
leafy tips			
raw	½ c	0.55 •	7
boiled, drained	½ c	0.54 •	10
pods			
raw	1 c	1.30 •	16
boiled, drained	½ c	0.65 •	12
bamboo shoots			
raw	½ c	0.53 •	21
boiled, drained	1 c	0.78 •	15
canned, drained solids	1 c	0.87 •	25

Fiber figures marked with • refer to *crude* fiber. Unmarked fiber figures refer to *dietary* fiber.

	Portion	Fiber (g)	Calories
basella *See* vinespinach, *below*			
beans, shellie, canned, solids & liquids	½ c	0.73 •	37
beans, snap			
raw	½ c	0.60 •	17
boiled, drained	½ c	0.89 •	22
canned			
solids & liquids	½ c	0.75 •	18
solids & liquids, seasoned	½ c	0.97 •	18
frozen, boiled, drained	½ c	0.70 •	18
beet greens			
raw	½ c	0.25 •	4
boiled, drained	½ c	0.72 •	20
beets			
raw	½ c sliced	0.54 •	30
boiled, drained	½ c sliced	0.76 •	26
canned, solids & liquids	½ c sliced	0.75 •	36
pickled, canned, solids & liquids	½ c	0.71 •	75
bittergourd; bittermelon *See* balsam pear, *above*			
bok choy *See* cabbage, Chinese, *below*			
borage			
raw	½ c	0.40 •	9
boiled, drained	3½ oz	1.07 •	25
broad beans *See* LEGUMES & LEGUME PRODUCTS			
broccoli			
raw	1 spear = 5.3 oz	1.68 •	42
boiled, drained	1 spear = 6.3 oz	2.16 •	53
	½ c	0.94 •	23
frozen, boiled, drained	½ c chopped	1.10 •	25
	½ c spears	2.78 •	69
	10 oz pkg spears	1.02 •	25
brussels sprouts			
boiled, drained	1 sprout = 0.73 oz	0.29 •	8
	½ c	1.07 •	30
frozen, boiled, drained	½ c	1.13 •	33
burdock root			
raw	1 c	2.29 •	85
	5½ oz	3.03 •	112

	Portion	Fiber (g)	Calories
boiled, drained	1 c	2.29 •	110
	5.8 oz	3.04 •	146
butterbur			
raw	1 c	1.22 •	13
boiled, drained	3½ oz	0.78 •	8
cabbage			
raw	½ c shredded	0.28 •	8
boiled, drained	½ c shredded	0.45 •	16
cabbage, Chinese			
bok choy			
raw	½ c shredded	0.21 •	5
boiled, drained	½ c shredded	0.51 •	10
pe-tsai			
raw	½ c shredded	0.23 •	6
boiled, drained	1 c shredded	0.60 •	16
cabbage, red			
raw	½ c shredded	0.35 •	10
boiled, drained	½ c shredded	0.57 •	16
cabbage, savoy			
raw	½ c shredded	0.28 •	10
boiled, drained	½ c shredded	0.51 •	18
carrots			
raw	½ c shredded	0.57 •	24
	2½ oz	0.75 •	31
boiled, drained	½ c sliced	1.15 •	35
	1.6 oz	0.68 •	21
canned			
drained solids	½ c sliced	0.58 •	17
solids & liquids	½ c sliced	0.91 •	28
frozen, boiled, drained	½ c sliced	0.86 •	26
cassava, raw	3½ oz	2.49 •	120
cauliflower			
raw	3 flowerets = 2 oz	0.47 •	13
	½ c pieces	0.42 •	12
boiled, drained	½ c pieces	0.51 •	15
frozen, boiled, drained	½ c pieces	0.72 •	17
celeriac			
raw	½ c	1.01 •	31
boiled, drained	3½ oz	0.83 •	25

Fiber figures marked with • refer to *crude* fiber. Unmarked fiber figures refer to *dietary* fiber.

	Portion	Fiber (g)	Calories
celery			
raw	1 stalk = 1.4 oz	0.28 •	6
	½ c diced	0.41 •	9
boiled, drained	½ c diced	0.49 •	11
celtuce, raw	1 leaf = 0.3 oz	0.03 •	2
chard, Swiss			
raw	½ c chopped	0.14 •	3
boiled, drained	½ c chopped	0.83 •	18
chayote, fruit			
raw	1 c pieces	0.92 •	32
	7.1 oz	1.42 •	49
boiled, drained	1 c pieces	0.93 •	38
chicory, raw			
greens	½ c chopped	0.72 •	21
roots	½ c pieces	0.88 •	33
Chinese parsley *See* coriander, *below*			
Chinese preserving melon *See* wax gourd, *below*			
chives			
raw	1 T	0.03 •	1
	1 t	0.01 •	0
freeze-dried	1 T	0.02 •	1
chrysanthemum, garland			
raw	1 c pieces	0.22 •	4
boiled, drained	½ c pieces	0.58 •	10
collards			
raw	½ c chopped	0.53 •	18
boiled, drained	½ c chopped	0.38 •	13
frozen, boiled, drained	½ c chopped	0.92 •	31
coriander (cilantro), raw	¼ c	0.03 •	1
corn, sweet			
raw	½ c kernels	0.54 •	66
	kernels from 1 ear	0.63 •	77
boiled, drained	½ c kernels	0.49 •	89
	kernels from 1 ear	0.46 •	83
canned			
cream style	½ c	0.62 •	93
in brine, solids & liquids	½ c	0.63 •	79
vacuum pack	½ c	0.82 •	83
w/red & green peppers, solids & liquids	½ c	0.71 •	86

	Portion	Fiber (g)	Calories
frozen, boiled, drained	½ c kernels	0.39 •	67
	kernels from 1 ear	0.41 •	59
cowpeas *See* LEGUMES & LEGUME PRODUCTS			
cress, garden			
raw	1 sprig	0.01 •	0
	½ c	0.28 •	8
boiled, drained	½ c	0.61 •	16
cucumber, raw	½ c sliced	0.31 •	7
	10½ oz	1.81 •	39
daikon *See* radishes: Oriental, *below*			
dandelion greens			
raw	½ c chopped	0.45 •	13
boiled, drained	½ c chopped	0.68 •	17
dasheen *See* taro, *below*			
dock			
raw	½ c chopped	0.54 •	15
boiled, drained	3½ oz	182	20
eggplant, boiled, drained	1 c cubed	0.47 •	27
endive, raw	½ c chopped	0.23 •	4
escarole *See* endive, *above*			
garlic, raw	1 clove = 0.1 oz	0.05 •	4
ginger root, raw	0.4 oz	0.11 •	8
	¼ c sliced	0.25 •	17
gourd			
dishcloth, boiled, drained	½ c sliced	0.34 •	50
white-flowered (calabash), boiled, drained	½ c cubed	0.46 •	11
horseradish-tree			
leafy tips			
raw	½ c chopped	0.15 •	6
boiled, drained	½ c chopped	0.36 •	13
pods			
raw	1 pod = 0.4 oz	0.14 •	4
boiled, drained	½ c sliced	1.09 •	21
hyacinth beans *See* LEGUMES & LEGUME PRODUCTS			
Jerusalem artichokes, raw	½ c sliced	0.6 •	57
jicama *See* yam bean, *below*			
jute (pot herb), boiled, drained	½ c	0.84 •	16

Fiber figures marked with • refer to *crude* fiber. Unmarked fiber figures refer to *dietary* fiber.

	Portion	Fiber (g)	Calories
kale			
raw	½ c chopped	0.51 •	17
boiled, drained	½ c chopped	0.52 •	21
frozen, boiled, drained	½ c chopped	0.60 •	20
kale, Scotch			
raw	½ c chopped	0.42 •	14
boiled, drained	½ c chopped	0.55 •	18
kanpyo (dried gourd strips)	0.7 oz	1.73 •	49
kohlrabi			
raw	½ c sliced	0.70 •	19
boiled, drained	½ c sliced	0.90 •	24
lamb's-quarters, boiled, drained	½ c chopped	1.62 •	29
leeks			
raw	¼ c chopped	0.39 •	16
boiled, drained	¼ c chopped	0.21 •	8
freeze-dried	1 T	0.02 •	1
lentils See LEGUMES & LEGUME PRODUCTS			
lettuce, raw			
cos or romaine	1 inner leaf = 0.35 oz	0.07 •	2
	½ c shredded	0.20 •	4
iceberg	1 leaf = 0.7 oz	0.11 •	3
	1 head = 1 lb 3 oz	2.86 •	70
looseleaf	1 leaf = 0.35 oz	0.07 •	2
	½ c shredded	0.20 •	5
lima beans See LEGUMES & LEGUME PRODUCTS			
lotus root, boiled, drained	3.1 oz	0.76 •	59
manioc See cassava, above			
mountain yam, Hawaii, steamed	½ c	0.40 •	59
mung beans See LEGUMES & LEGUME PRODUCTS			
mushrooms			
raw	½ c pieces	0.26 •	9
boiled, drained	½ c pieces	0.68 •	21
mushrooms, shitake			
cooked	½ oz	1.41 •	40
dried	0.1 oz	0.41 •	11
mustard greens			
raw	½ c chopped	0.31 •	7
boiled, drained	½ c chopped	0.48 •	11
frozen, boiled, drained	½ c chopped	0.55 •	14
mustard spinach			
raw	½ c chopped	0.75 •	17

	Portion	Fiber (g)	Calories
boiled, drained	½ c chopped	0.72 •	14
New Zealand spinach			
raw	½ c chopped	0.20 •	4
boiled, drained	½ c chopped	0.55 •	11
okra			
boiled, drained	½ c sliced	0.72 •	25
frozen, boiled, drained	½ c sliced	0.94 •	34
onions			
raw	1 T chopped	0.04 •	3
	½ c chopped	0.35 •	27
boiled, drained	1 T chopped	0.06 •	4
	½ c chopped	0.44 •	29
dehydrated flakes	1 T	0.23 •	16
frozen, boiled, drained	1 T chopped	0.07 •	4
	½ c chopped	0.48 •	30
onions, spring, raw	1 T chopped	0.05 •	2
	½ c chopped	0.42 •	13
onions, Welsh, raw	3½ oz	1.00 •	34
oysterplant *See* salsify, *below*			
parsley			
raw	10 sprigs = 0.35 oz	0.12 •	3
	½ c chopped	0.36 •	10
freeze-dried	1 T	0.04 •	1
parsnips			
raw	½ c sliced	1.34 •	50
boiled, drained	½ c sliced	1.72 •	63
peas & carrots			
canned, solids & liquids	½ c	1.46 •	48
frozen, boiled, drained	½ c	1.11 •	38
	10 oz pkg	3.86 •	133
peas & onions, canned, solids & liquids	½ c	0.74 •	30
peas, edible pods			
raw	½ c	1.80 •	30
boiled, drained	½ c	0.83 •	34
frozen, boiled, drained	½ c	2.40 •	42
	10 oz pkg	7.61 •	132
peas, green			
raw	½ c	1.72 •	63
boiled, drained	½ c	1.85 •	67

Fiber figures marked with • refer to *crude* fiber. Unmarked fiber figures refer to *dietary* fiber.

	Portion	Fiber (g)	Calories
peas, green *(cont.)*			
canned			
drained solids	½ c	1.69 •	59
solids & liquids	½ c	1.77 •	61
solids & liquids, seasoned	½ c	1.93 •	57
frozen, boiled, drained	½ c	1.71 •	63
peas, mature seeds, sprouted, raw	½ c	1.67 •	77
peas, split *See* split peas, *under* LEGUMES & LEGUME PRODUCTS			
pepeao			
raw	0.2 oz	0.13 •	2
dried	½ c	3.71 •	36
peppers			
hot chili			
raw	1 pepper = 1.6 oz	0.81 •	18
	½ c chopped	1.35 •	30
canned, solids & liquids	1 pepper = 2.6 oz	0.88 •	18
	½ c chopped	0.82 •	17
jalapeño, canned, solids & liquids	½ c chopped	1.56 •	17
sweet			
raw	1 pepper = 2.6 oz	0.89 •	18
	½ c chopped	0.60 •	12
boiled, drained	1 pepper = 2.6 oz	0.64 •	13
	½ c chopped	0.60 •	12
canned, solids & liquids	½ c halves	0.56 •	13
freeze-dried	1 T	0.07 •	1
	¼ c	0.26 •	5
frozen, boiled, drained	3½ oz chopped	0.88 •	18
frozen, unprepared, chopped	10 oz pkg	2.84 •	58
pigeon peas *See* LEGUMES & LEGUME PRODUCTS			
pinto beans *See* LEGUMES & LEGUME PRODUCTS			
poi	½ c	0.65 •	134
potatoes			
raw			
flesh	3.9 oz	0.49 •	88
skin	1.3 oz	0.68 •	22
baked			
flesh & skin	7.1 oz	1.33 •	220
flesh	5½ oz	0.59 •	145
skin	2 oz	1.32 •	115

	Portion	Fiber (g)	Calories
boiled in skin			
flesh	4.8 oz	0.43 •	119
skin	1.2 oz	1.25 •	27
boiled w/out skin, flesh	4.8 oz	0.51 •	116
canned			
drained solids	1.2 oz	0.09 •	21
solids & liquids	1 c	0.71 •	120
frozen, whole, unprepared	½ c	0.36 •	71
microwaved in skin			
flesh & skin	7.1 oz	1.64 •	212
flesh	5½ oz	0.64 •	156
skin	2 oz	1.79 •	77
pumpkin			
boiled, drained	½ c mashed	1.01 •	24
canned	½ c	1.97 •	41
pumpkin flowers			
raw	1 c	0.21 •	5
boiled, drained	½ c	0.62 •	10
pumpkin leaves, boiled, drained	½ c	0.37 •	7
purslane			
raw	1 c	0.93 •	7
boiled, drained	1 c	0.34 •	21
radishes, raw	10 radishes = 1.6 oz	0.24 •	7
Oriental			
raw	½ c	0.28 •	8
boiled, drained	½ c sliced	0.36 •	13
dried	½ c	4.85 •	157
white icicle, raw	½ c sliced	0.35 •	7
rutabagas			
raw	½ c cubed	0.77 •	25
boiled, drained	½ c cubed	0.89 •	29
	½ c mashed	1.25 •	41
salsify			
raw	½ c sliced	1.21 •	55
boiled, drained	½ c sliced	1.01 •	46
seaweed			
agar, raw	3½ oz	0.45 •	26
kelp, raw	3½ oz	1.33 •	43
laver, raw	3½ oz	0.27 •	35

Fiber figures marked with • refer to *crude* fiber. Unmarked fiber figures refer to *dietary* fiber.

	Portion	Fiber (g)	Calories
seaweed *(cont.)*			
spirulina			
raw	3½ oz	0.34 •	26
dried	3½ oz	3.64 •	290
wakame, raw	3½ oz	0.54 •	45
sesbania flower			
raw	1 c	0.30 •	5
steamed	1 c	1.61 •	23
shallots			
raw	1 T chopped	0.07 •	7
freeze-dried	1 T	0.04 •	3
snow peas *See* peas, edible pods, *above*			
soybeans *See* SOYBEANS & SOYBEAN PRODUCTS			
spinach			
raw	½ c chopped	0.25 •	6
boiled, drained	½ c	0.79 •	21
canned, solids & liquids	½ c	0.80 •	22
frozen, boiled, drained	½ c	1.04 •	27
	10 oz pkg	2.42 •	63
spinach, mustard *See* mustard spinach, *above*			
spinach, New Zealand *See* New Zealand spinach, *above*			
split peas *See* LEGUMES & LEGUME PRODUCTS			
sprouts *See plant name (alfalfa, mung bean, etc.)*			
squash, summer			
crookneck			
raw	½ c sliced	0.36 •	12
boiled, drained	½ c sliced	0.54 •	18
canned, drained solids	½ c sliced	0.41 •	14
frozen, boiled, drained	½ c sliced	0.78 •	24
scallop			
raw	½ c sliced	0.36 •	12
boiled, drained	½ c sliced	0.43 •	14
zucchini			
raw	½ c sliced	0.29 •	9
boiled, drained	½ c sliced	0.45 •	14
canned, Italian style, in tomato sauce	½ c	0.58 •	33
frozen, boiled, drained	½ c	0.62 •	19
other varieties			
raw	½ c sliced	0.39 •	13
boiled, drained	½ c sliced	0.54 •	18
squash, winter			
acorn			
baked	½ c cubed	2.00 •	57
boiled	½ c mashed	1.44 •	41

	Portion	Fiber (g)	Calories
butternut			
baked	½ c cubed	1.28 •	41
frozen, boiled	½ c mashed	1.04 •	47
hubbard			
baked	½ c cubed	1.77 •	51
boiled	½ c mashed	1.22 •	35
spaghetti, boiled, drained, baked	½ c	1.09 •	23
other varieties			
raw	½ c cubed	0.81 •	21
baked	½ c cubed	0.72 •	39
string beans See beans, snap, above			
succotash			
boiled, drained	½ c	1.29 •	111
canned			
w/whole kernel corn, solids & liquids	½ c	0.79 •	81
w/cream-style corn	½ c	1.71 •	102
frozen, boiled, drained	½ c	0.87 •	79
swamp cabbage			
raw	1 c chopped	0.62 •	11
boiled, drained	1 c chopped	0.83 •	20
sweet potato leaves			
raw	1 c chopped	0.42 •	12
steamed	1 c	0.84 •	22
sweet potatoes			
baked in skin	1 potato = 4 oz	0.91 •	118
	½ c mashed	0.80 •	103
boiled w/out skin	½ c mashed	1.39 •	172
candied	3.7 oz	0.41 •	144
canned			
vacuum packed	1 c mashed	1.80 •	233
	1 c pieces	1.41 •	183
in syrup, drained solids	1 c	1.10 •	213
in syrup, solids & liquids	1 c	1.05 •	202
frozen, baked	½ c cubed	0.68 •	88
Swiss chard See chard, Swiss, above			
taro			
raw	½ c sliced	0.42 •	56
cooked	½ c sliced	0.57 •	94

Fiber figures marked with • refer to *crude* fiber. Unmarked fiber figures refer to *dietary* fiber.

	Portion	Fiber (g)	Calories
taro chips	10 chips = 0.8 oz	0.27 •	110
taro leaves			
raw	1 c	0.57 •	12
steamed	1 c	0.78 •	35
taro shoots			
raw	1 shoot = 2.9 oz	0.48 •	9
cooked	½ c sliced	0.38 •	10
taro, Tahitian			
raw	½ c sliced	1.09 •	25
cooked	½ c sliced	1.55 •	30
tomatoes, green, raw	1 tomato = 4.3 oz	0.62 •	30
tomatoes, red, ripe			
raw	1 tomato = 4.3 oz	0.57 •	24
boiled	½ c	0.92 •	30
canned			
whole	½ c	0.55 •	24
stewed	½ c	0.54 •	34
wedges in juice	½ c	0.58 •	34
w/green chilies	½ c	0.42 •	18
stewed	1 c	0.48 •	59
tomato paste, canned	½ c	1.25 •	110
tomato puree, canned	1 c	2.05 •	102
tomato sauce *See* SAUCES & GRAVIES			
towel gourd *See* gourd: dishcloth, *above*			
tree fern, cooked	½ c chopped	0.43 •	28
turnip greens			
raw	½ c chopped	0.22 •	7
boiled, drained	½ c chopped	0.44 •	15
canned, solids & liquids	½ c	0.71 •	17
frozen, boiled, drained	½ c	0.85 •	24
turnip greens & turnips, frozen, boiled, drained	3½ oz	0.52 •	17
turnips			
raw	½ c cubed	0.59 •	18
boiled, drained	½ c cubed	0.55 •	14
frozen, boiled, drained	3½ oz	0.68 •	23
vegetables, mixed			
canned			
drained solids	½ c	1.07 •	39
solids & liquids	½ c	1.46 •	44
frozen, boiled, drained	½ c	1.07 •	54
	10 oz pkg	3.22 •	163

	Portion	Fiber (g)	Calories
vinespinach, raw	3½ oz	0.70 •	19
water chestnuts, Chinese			
raw	1¼ oz	0.29 •	38
canned, solids & liquids	1 oz	0.16 •	14
watercress, raw	½ c chopped	0.12 •	2
wax beans *See* beans, snap, *above*			
wax gourd (Chinese preserving melon), boiled, drained	½ c cubed	0.44 •	11
winged beans *See* LEGUMES & LEGUME PRODUCTS			
yam bean (tuber only)			
raw	1 c sliced	0.84 •	49
boiled, drained	3½ oz	1.12 •	46
yardlong beans *See* LEGUMES & LEGUME PRODUCTS			

Vegetables, Prepared

	Portion	Fiber (g)	Calories
coleslaw	½ c	0.36 •	42
corn pudding	1 c	0.90 •	271
onion rings, breaded, frozen, heated in oven	0.7 oz	0.08 •	81
potato chips *See* SNACKS			
potato pancakes, homemade	2.7 oz	0.50 •	495
potato puffs, frozen, fried in vegetable oil	¼ oz	0.04 •	16
potato salad	½ c	0.46 •	179
potatoes, au gratin			
dry mix, prepared	5½ oz pkg	1.40 •	764
homemade	½ c	0.33 •	160
potatoes, french fried, frozen			
cottage-cut, heated in oven	1.8 oz	0.36 •	109
extruded, heated in oven	1.8 oz	0.35 •	163
fried in animal fat & vegetable oil	1.8 oz	0.37 •	158
fried in vegetable oil	1.8 oz	0.37 •	158
heated in oven	1.8 oz	0.34 •	111
potatoes, hashed brown			
frozen, plain, prepared	½ c	0.42 •	170
homemade, prepared in vegetable oil	½ c	0.32 •	163

Fiber figures marked with • refer to *crude* fiber. Unmarked fiber figures refer to *dietary* fiber.

	Portion	Fiber (g)	Calories
potatoes, mashed			
dehydrated flakes, prepared, whole milk & butter added	½ c	0.50 •	118
granules w/milk, prepared	½ c	0.32 •	83
homemade w/whole milk	½ c	0.33 •	81
homemade w/whole milk & margarine	½ c	0.32 •	111
potatoes, O'Brien			
homemade	1 c	0.83 •	157
potatoes, scalloped			
dry mix, prepared w/whole milk & 5½ oz pkg	2.22 •	764	
homemade	½ c	0.36 •	105
sauerkraut, canned, solids & liquids	½ c	1.26 •	22
spinach soufflé	1 c	0.81 •	218

▪ BRAND NAME

B&B
| mushrooms, canned | 2 oz | 0.8 | 25 |

Birds Eye Frozen Vegetables
CHEESE SAUCE COMBINATION

baby brussels sprouts w/cheese sauce	4½ oz	2.4	110
broccoli w/cheese sauce	5 oz	2.1	120
broccoli w/creamy Italian cheese sauce	4½ oz	2.2	90
cauliflower w/cheese sauce	5 oz	1.2	110
peas & pearl onions w/cheese sauce	5 oz	2.9	140

COMBINATION

broccoli, carrots, pasta twists	3.3 oz	1.4	90
corn, green beans, pasta curls	3.3 oz	1.6	110
creamed spinach	3 oz	1.4	60
green peas & pearl onions	3.3 oz	3.4	70
green peas & potatoes w/cream sauce	2.6 oz	1.7	130
mixed vegetables w/onion sauce	2.6 oz	1.3	100

	Portion	Fiber (g)	Calories
DELUXE			
beans, whole green	3 oz	1.8	25
carrots, baby peas, & pearl onions	3.3 oz	1.9	50
carrots, whole baby	3.3 oz	1.4	40
corn, tender sweet	3.3 oz	2.3	80
peas, tender tiny	3.3 oz	3.5	60
FARM FRESH MIXTURES			
broccoli, baby carrots, water chestnuts	3.2 oz	3.0	35
broccoli, cauliflower, carrots	3.2 oz	3.0	25
broccoli, corn, red peppers	3.2 oz	3.0	50
broccoli, green beans, pearl onions, red peppers	3.2 oz	3.0	25
broccoli, red peppers, bamboo shoots, straw mushrooms	3.2 oz	3.0	25
brussels sprouts, cauliflower, carrots	3.2 oz	4.0	30
cauliflower, baby whole carrots, snow pea pods	3.2 oz	3.0	30
INTERNATIONAL RECIPES			
Bavarian style	3.3 oz	1.6	110
Chinese style	3.3 oz	0.8	80
chow mein style	3.3 oz	1.0	90
Italian style	3.3 oz	0.9	110
Japanese style	3.3 oz	1.5	100
Mandarin style	3.3 oz	0.5	90
New England style	3.3 oz	1.7	130
pasta primavera style	3.3 oz	1.5	120
San Francisco style	3.3 oz	1.2	100
REGULAR			
beans			
cut or French cut green	3 oz	2.1	25
Italian green	3 oz	2.6	30

Fiber figures marked with • refer to *crude* fiber. Unmarked fiber figures refer to *dietary* fiber.

	Portion	Fiber (g)	Calories
broccoli			
chopped	3.3 oz	2.8	25
cuts	3.3 oz	2.6	25
brussels sprouts	3.3 oz	3.3	35
cauliflower	3.3 oz	1.5	25
corn, sweet	3.3 oz	2.3	80
mixed vegetables	3.3 oz	2.4	60
peas, green	3.3 oz	4.4	80
spinach			
whole leaf	3.3 oz	2.8	20
chopped	3.3 oz	2.7	20
squash, cooked, winter	4 oz	1.5	45
STIR-FRY			
Chinese style	3.3 oz	1.4	35
Japanese style	3.3 oz	1.3	30
Joan of Arc			
garden salad	½ c	2.4	70
potato salad			
German style	½ c	1.6	120
Home Style	½ c	1.5	170
yams			
whole, packed in heavy syrup	½ c	2.1	120
mashed	½ c	2	90
in orange pineapple sauce	½ c	2	190
Le Sueur			
FROZEN, IN BUTTER SAUCE			
early peas	½ c	4.9	70
minipeas, pea pods, & water chestnuts	½ c	3	80
peas, carrots, & onions	½ c	3	80
Mexicorn			
Mexicorn w/peppers	½ c	3	80
Pillsbury			
BUTTER SAUCE VEGETABLES			
baby lima beans	½ c	4	110
broccoli spears	½ c	2	45
brussels sprouts	½ c	2	40
cut green beans	½ c	1.5	30
cut leaf spinach	½ c	3.5	45
French-style green beans	½ c	2	35
mixed vegetables	½ c	2	70
Niblets corn	½ c	2	100
sweet peas	½ c	4	80

	Portion	Fiber (g)	Calories
CANNED VEGETABLES			
asparagus cuts/spears	½ c	1.2	20
cream-style corn	½ c	3.5	100
cut green beans	½ c	1.2	20
mushrooms	½ c	1.3	25
mushrooms in butter sauce	2 oz	0.6	30
sweet peas	½ c	4.8	50
sweet peas & onions	½ c	4	50
three bean salad	½ c	1.5	70
whole kernel corn, vacuum pack	½ c	2.6	80
CREAM & CHEESE SAUCE COMBINATION			
baby brussels sprouts in cheese-flavored sauce	½ c	2.8	70
broccoli cauliflower carrots in cheese-flavored sauce	½ c	· 2	70
broccoli in cheese-flavored sauce	½ c	2	60
broccoli in white cheddar cheese–flavored sauce	½ c	2	50
cauliflower in cheese-flavored sauce	½ c	2.4	60
cauliflower in white cheddar cheese–flavored sauce	½ c	2	50
cream-style corn	½ c	2	110
creamed spinach	½ c	0.6	80
peas in cream sauce	½ c	3.5	90
HARVEST FRESH			
broccoli spears	½ c	2.4	20
cut broccoli	½ c	2	18
cut green beans	½ c	1.7	16
early June peas	½ c	3.3	60
lima beans	½ c	5.2	60
mixed vegetables	½ c	2.5	45
Niblets corn	½ c	3	80
spinach	½ c	2.8	25
sweet peas	½ c	3.4	50

Fiber figures marked with • refer to *crude* fiber. Unmarked fiber figures refer to *dietary* fiber.

	Portion	Fiber (g)	Calories
POLYBAG VEGETABLES			
broccoli cuts	½ c	2	12
brussels sprouts	½ c	2.6	25
cauliflower cuts	½ c	1.4	12
green beans	½ c	1.5	14
lima beans	½ c	5	100
mixed vegetables	½ c	2.3	50
Niblets corn	½ c	1.7	80
Niblets corn on the cob	1 ear	3	150
sweet peas	½ c	3.5	50
VALLEY COMBINATION DUAL POUCH W/SAUCE			
American-style vegetables	½ c	3.4	70
Broccoli Cauliflower Medley	½ c	3	50
Broccoli Fanfare	½ c	2.9	70
Italian-style vegetables	½ c	2.8	40
Japanese-style vegetables	½ c	2.9	45
Le Sueur–style vegetables	½ c	5.2	60
Mexican-style vegetables	½ c	4.2	140
VALLEY COMBINATIONS, POLYBAG			
Broccoli Carrot Fanfare	½ c	2.1	20
Broccoli Cauliflower Supreme	½ c	2.1	20
Cauliflower Green Bean Festival	½ c	2	16
Corn Broccoli Bounty	½ c	1.9	45
Sweet Pea Cauliflower Medley	½ c	2.5	30

❑ **YOGURT** *See* **MILK, MILK SUBSTITUTES, & MILK PRODUCTS**